METABOLIC CONFUSION DIET

FOOD LIST FOR ENDOMORPH WOMEN

Unlock Your Body's Potential with Foods and a 28-Day Meal Plan Tailored for Optimal Health and Weight Loss through Healthy Eating to Boost Metabolism.

MARTHA J. KELVIN

Disclaimer:
The information provided in this book, is intended for educational purposes only. It is not a substitute for professional medical advice, diagnosis, or treatment. Always seek the advice of your physician or other qualified healthcare provider with any questions you may have regarding a medical condition.

The author and publisher of this book have made every effort to ensure that the information provided is accurate and up-to-date at the time of publication. However, medical knowledge and research are constantly evolving, and information may become outdated or subject to change. Therefore, the author and publisher do not warrant or guarantee the accuracy, completeness, or timeliness of the information presented in this book.

The author and publisher shall not be liable for any direct or indirect damages or injuries arising out of the use, interpretation, or application of any information provided in this book. Readers are encouraged to consult with their healthcare providers for individualized advice and recommendations based on their specific medical conditions and needs.

By reading this book, you acknowledge and agree to the terms of this disclaimer.
Printed in the United States of America.

First Edition: February 2024

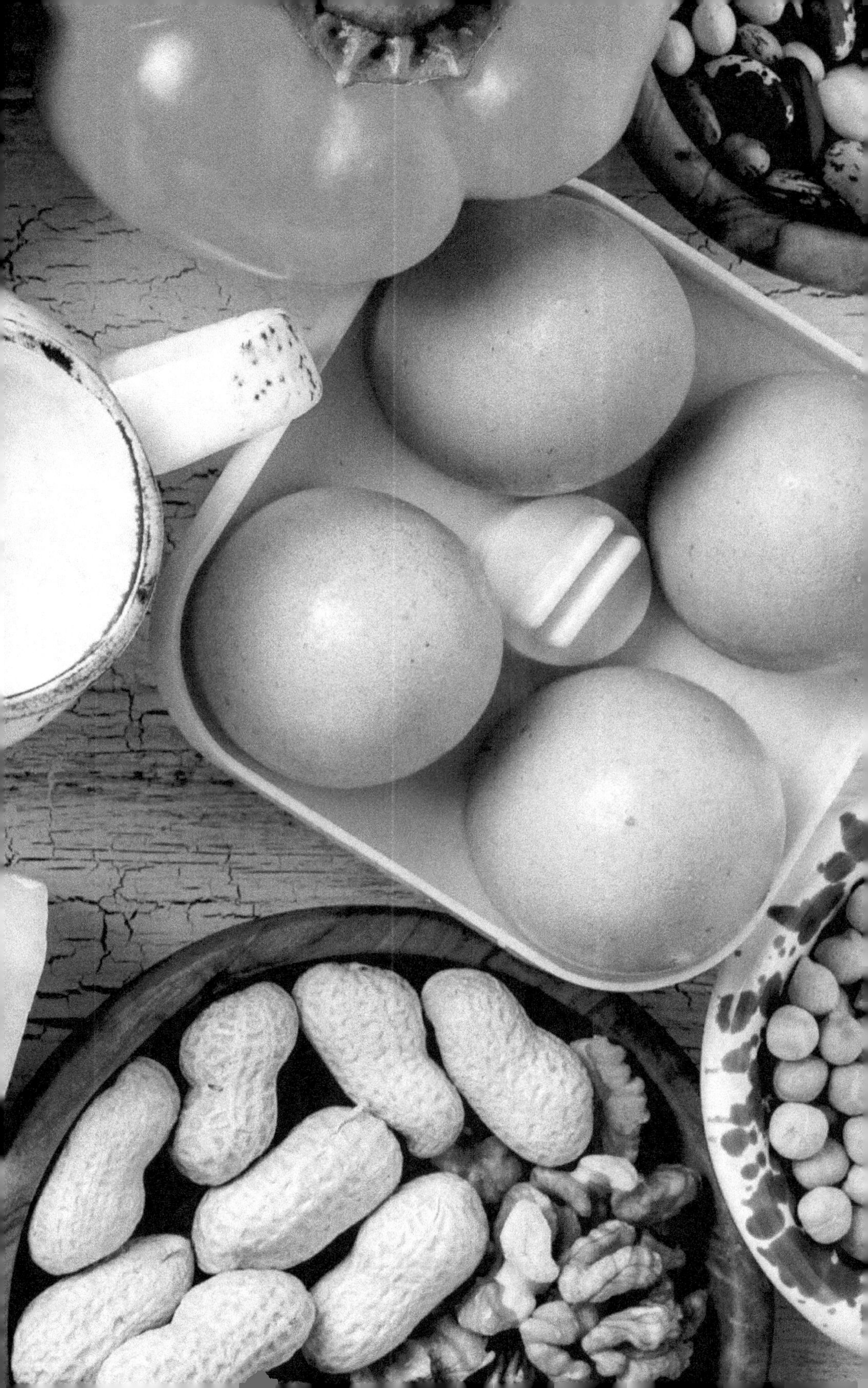

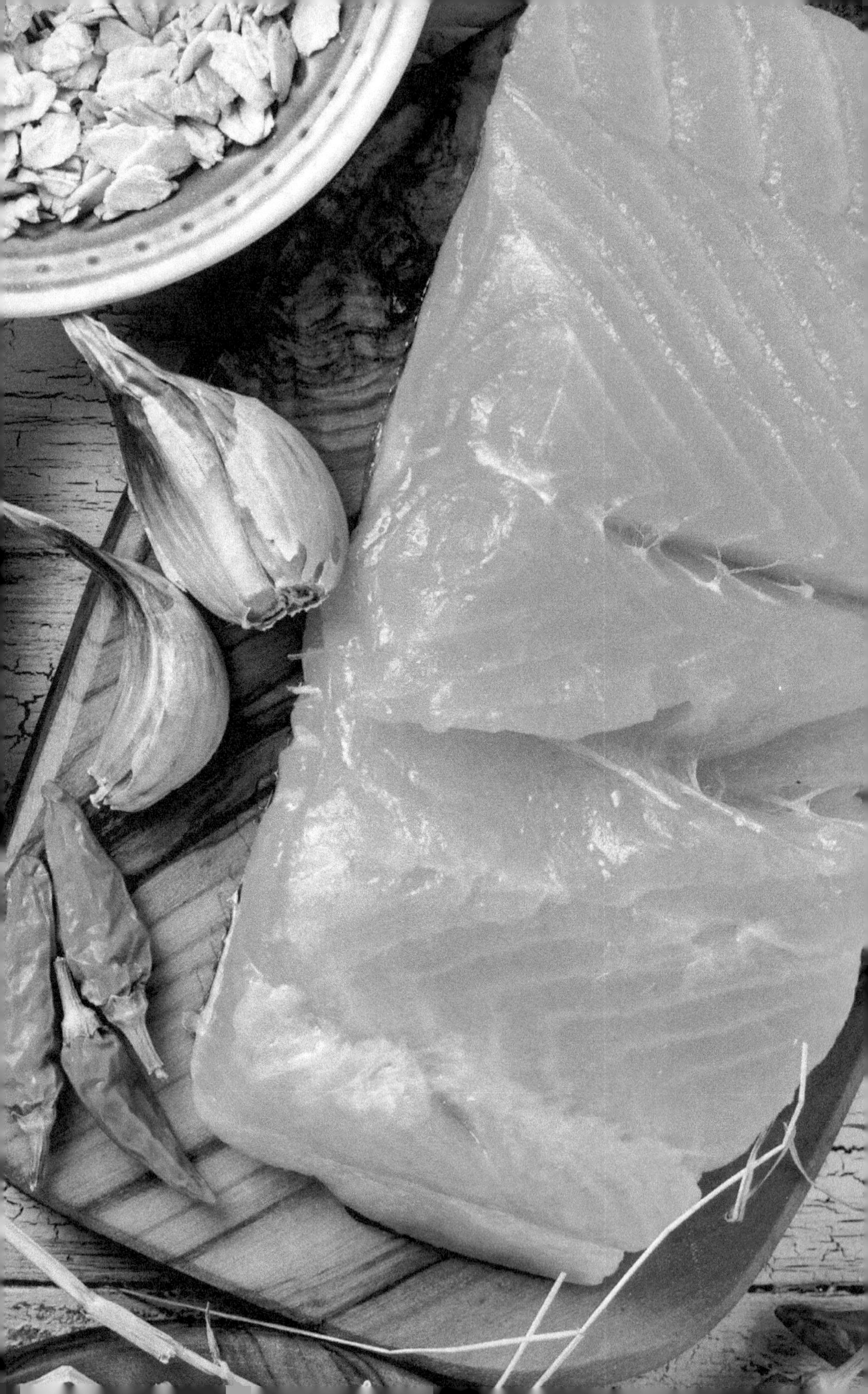

CONTENTS

INTRODUCTION

Welcome to "Metabolic Confusion Diet Food List for Endomorph Women"! If you've found yourself on this page, chances are, you're on a quest to understand your body better, seeking ways to navigate the often confusing world of dieting, or simply looking for a sustainable path to achieve your health and fitness goals. You're in the right place, and we're here to embark on this journey together.

First off, let's address the elephant in the room—dieting is no one-size-fits-all affair. Especially for us endomorph women, the traditional diet advice that seems to work wonders for others can often leave us feeling stuck, frustrated, and downright disheartened. It's like our bodies have a mind of their own, holding onto every calorie like a treasure, making weight loss feel like an uphill battle.

But here's the good news: it's not your fault, and there's a way forward that doesn't involve drastic fasting or cutting out entire food groups. Enter the concept of metabolic confusion—a diet strategy that promises to kickstart your metabolism into high gear, encouraging your body to burn fat more efficiently without feeling deprived or hitting those dreaded plateaus. Sounds intriguing, right?

Metabolic confusion isn't about tricking your body per se but rather about optimizing your metabolism through varying caloric intake. It's about saying goodbye to the monotony of eating the same calorie-restricted meals day in and day out, and hello to a dynamic eating plan that keeps your body guessing—and burning.

Now, you might be thinking, "That sounds great, but where do I start? What foods should I eat? How do I apply this to my life as an endomorph woman?" These are all valid questions, and this book is designed to answer each one of them, guiding you through the process with ease and confidence.

As an endomorph, your body is beautifully efficient at storing energy, which is a blessing in times of scarcity but a challenge in our modern world of abundance. This book will help you understand your body type better, acknowledging its strengths and how to work with its tendencies, rather than against them. You'll learn that the key to unlocking your metabolic potential doesn't lie in perpetual restriction but in understanding and harnessing the power of food to work for you, not against you.

We'll dive deep into the principles of metabolic confusion, laying out a clear, actionable plan that includes high-calorie and low-calorie phases. But don't worry, this isn't about bingeing and starving. It's a carefully structured approach that ensures you get the nutrients your body needs to thrive while also promoting fat loss and preventing metabolic stagnation.

The core of this book is the comprehensive food list tailored specifically for endomorph women. We'll cover proteins, carbohydrates, fats, vegetables, fruits, and even beverages, giving you the tools to create meals that satisfy, nourish, and support your metabolic goals. You'll find that this diet isn't just about weight loss;

it's about empowering you to make informed choices that enhance your overall health and wellbeing.

But what's knowledge without application? That's why we've included sample meal plans that illustrate how to incorporate these foods into your daily life, making the metabolic confusion diet a practical, achievable lifestyle, not just another fad. Plus, we'll explore the crucial role of exercise, supplements, and how to track your progress, ensuring you have a holistic approach to reaching your goals.

This journey is about more than just shedding pounds; it's about gaining a deeper understanding and appreciation for your body, learning to nourish it in a way that promotes health, vitality, and happiness. It's about breaking free from the cycle of restrictive dieting and embracing a way of eating that's dynamic, satisfying, and, most importantly, effective.

So, whether you're a seasoned dieter tired of the same old routines or someone just starting to explore the world of nutrition and fitness, this book is for you. It's a testament to the fact that with the right knowledge and tools, achieving your health and fitness goals is not only possible but enjoyable.

As we embark on this journey together, remember: you're not alone. Countless women share your struggles and your aspirations. This book is a gathering of collective wisdom, a guide created to support you, inspire you, and empower you to take control of your health in a way that celebrates your unique body.

So, let's turn the page and begin this exciting adventure towards understanding, transforming, and loving your endomorph body. Welcome to the metabolic confusion diet for endomorph women. Welcome to a new beginning.

INTRODUCTION TO METABOLIC CONFUSION

Understanding Metabolic Confusion

Metabolic confusion sounds like a complex term, right? But at its heart, it's about bringing a delightful variety into your diet. It's like when you shuffle your playlist because you're tired of hearing the same tunes over and over. Your body, much like you with your music, craves variety to stay engaged and lively. This strategy is about giving your metabolism little surprises that keep it guessing and, more importantly, burning fat more effectively.

Now, let's talk about how this whole thing works. Think of your body as this incredibly smart, adaptive system. Feed it the same amount of calories day in and day out, and it'll adapt, becoming super-efficient with those calories. Handy for survival, but not so much when you're trying to lose weight. This is where metabolic confusion steps in, like a friend who suggests an impromptu road trip to break the monotony of everyday life. On some days, you'll fuel up with more calories, telling your metabolism, "Party's on!" On other days, you'll dial it back, and your body, still in party mode, will turn to its fat stores for energy.

But here's a crucial nugget of truth: metabolic confusion isn't a free pass to indulge on high-calorie days, nor is it about starving yourself on low-calorie days. It's more like a balanced dance, where you're mindful of both the steps and the rhythm, ensuring your body gets the right mix of nutrients while also encouraging it to burn fat.

For those of us with endomorph bodies, this method whispers promise. Our bodies tend to cling to fat with a tenacity that's admirable but, frankly, a bit frustrating when we're trying to lose weight. Metabolic confusion offers a way to gently coax our metabolism into being a bit more generous, helping us shed those stubborn pounds.

Now, if you're wondering whether this will leave you feeling starved or overfed, let me ease your mind. This approach is all about balance and sustainability. It's designed to fit seamlessly into your life, making you feel nourished and satisfied, not deprived or overstuffed. It's about finding joy in the foods you eat and peace with the way your body looks and feels.

Metabolic confusion is more than just a diet trick; it's a new way to view your relationship with food and your body. It's about ending the war with your weight and starting a dialogue, learning to understand and work with your body's natural rhythms. It's a journey towards balance, where dieting doesn't mean deprivation, and being healthy doesn't mean being hungry.

Benefits of Metabolic Confusion for Endomorph Women

Embarking on the journey of metabolic confusion, especially for us endomorph women, is like discovering a secret path in a dense forest—a path that leads to a clearing filled with sunlight, where the struggles with weight management and metabolism seem far less daunting. This chapter is dedicated to unveiling the benefits of metabolic confusion for endomorph women, shedding light on how this approach can be a transformative tool in our health and fitness endeavors.

A Tailored Approach for Endomorphs

First, let's understand why metabolic confusion feels like it's tailor-made for endomorph body types. Our bodies, with their remarkable efficiency in storing fat and slow metabolism, often react stubbornly to conventional dieting methods. The metabolic confusion diet, with its rhythmic alteration between calorie intake levels, seems to speak directly to our metabolic sensitivities. It's like having a key to a previously unopenable door, offering us a way to communicate with our bodies more effectively.

Breaking through Plateaus

One of the most significant benefits of metabolic confusion for endomorph women is its potential to break through weight loss plateaus. These plateaus are not just physical barriers but emotional ones, often leading to frustration and demotivation. By varying our calorie intake, we keep our metabolism guessing, preventing it from settling into a comfortable routine and slowing down. This constant metabolic stimulation can lead to consistent weight loss, turning those plateaus into mere stepping stones.

Enhanced Fat Burning

Metabolic confusion can shift the body's energy utilization from relying heavily on carbohydrates to tapping into fat stores for energy. On lower calorie days, when the intake of energy is reduced, the body is encouraged to burn fat for fuel. This shift not only aids in weight loss but also in the reduction of body fat percentage, a critical factor in improving overall health and body composition.

Improved Relationship with Food

Dieting, for many, is synonymous with restriction and deprivation. However, metabolic confusion introduces a refreshing perspective by incorporating high-calorie days. These days allow for more flexibility and the inclusion of a wider variety of foods, which can prevent the common pitfall of binge eating associated with strict dieting. It fosters a healthier relationship with food, where eating becomes a joyous activity rather than a source of stress.

Sustainable Weight Management

The beauty of metabolic confusion lies in its sustainability. Unlike extreme diets that are difficult to maintain over time, metabolic confusion is a balanced approach. It doesn't cut out food groups or require drastic changes that are hard to stick with. This sustainability is crucial for long-term weight management and health, making it a practical choice for endomorph women looking for lasting results.

Boosted Energy Levels

Fluctuating calorie intake can also lead to improved energy levels. On high-calorie days, the body receives an influx of energy, which can fuel more intense workouts. On low-calorie days, the body's efficiency in using fat as fuel can keep energy levels steady, preventing the dips associated with constant calorie restriction. This balance can make it easier to stay active and engaged in your fitness journey.

Hormonal Balance

Dieting can sometimes wreak havoc on our hormonal balance, affecting everything from our mood to our metabolism. The metabolic confusion approach, by preventing extreme calorie restriction, can help maintain a healthier hormonal profile. This balance is crucial for weight loss, as hormones play a significant role in regulating appetite, fat distribution, and metabolism.

Enhanced Metabolic Flexibility

Metabolic confusion can improve the body's metabolic flexibility—the ability to switch between burning carbs and fats for energy efficiently. This flexibility is not just beneficial for weight loss but also for overall metabolic health, reducing the risk of insulin resistance and diabetes. For endomorph women, who may struggle with these issues, improving metabolic flexibility is a significant step towards better health.

Mental and Emotional Well-being

Let's not overlook the mental and emotional benefits. The sense of control and progress that comes with a successful metabolic confusion approach can be a powerful boost to self-esteem and mental health.

When weight loss becomes a journey of discovery rather than a battle, it can lead to a more positive body image and a deeper appreciation for what our bodies are capable of.

Customizability and Flexibility

Finally, metabolic confusion is highly customizable. You can adjust your high and low-calorie days based on your lifestyle, preferences, and goals. This flexibility ensures that the diet fits into your life, not the other way around. Whether you're a busy mom, a career woman, or juggling multiple roles, you can tailor metabolic confusion to suit your needs, making it a practical choice for real-life challenges.

How Metabolic Confusion Can Help Overcome Weight Loss Plateaus

Embarking on a weight loss journey can often feel like setting sail on unpredictable seas. You start with clear skies and smooth sailing, witnessing the pounds drop as you adhere to a new eating plan. However, as many of us have experienced, there comes a point where the waters become eerily calm, and despite your best efforts, the scale refuses to budge. This, my friends, is the dreaded weight loss plateau. But fear not, for metabolic confusion offers a lifeline, a way to navigate through these stagnant waters and get back on course toward your weight loss goals.

Understanding Weight Loss Plateaus

Before we delve into the solution, let's understand the problem. A weight loss plateau is a period where there is no significant change in body weight despite continuing with dieting and exercise efforts. It's a common phenomenon that can be incredibly frustrating. The human body is remarkably adaptable; when you reduce your calorie intake, your body eventually adjusts to this new level of energy intake, slowing down your metabolism to conserve energy. It's the body's survival mechanism kicking in, but unfortunately, it can make weight loss much more challenging.

Enter Metabolic Confusion

Metabolic confusion, with its approach of varying calorie intake, offers a strategic way to trick the body out of this conservation mode. By alternating between higher-calorie and lower-calorie periods, you prevent your body from adapting to a single, constant caloric intake. This variation can reinvigorate your metabolism, encouraging your body to continue burning fat instead of plateauing.

The Mechanism behind Metabolic Confusion

1. **Breaking the Adaptation Cycle**: Our bodies are designed to adapt to consistent conditions. By regularly changing your calorie intake, you're essentially keeping your body guessing, preventing it from settling into the energy-conservation mode that can cause plateaus.

2. **Stimulating Metabolism**: On higher-calorie days, you're essentially sending a signal to your metabolism that there's plenty of energy available, encouraging it to ramp up. This can lead to increased calorie burn, even on days when you're consuming less.

3. **Preserving Muscle Mass**: One risk of continuous low-calorie dieting is muscle loss, which in turn can slow down metabolism since muscle burns more calories than fat. The higher-calorie periods of metabolic confusion help provide the nutrients needed to maintain and even build muscle, supporting a healthier metabolism.

4. **Psychological Benefits**: Let's not underestimate the power of mental and emotional well-being in our weight loss journey. Metabolic confusion, with its built-in variety, can prevent the boredom and dietary fatigue that come with strict, monotonous eating plans. This variety can keep you motivated and less likely to give up on your diet.

Implementing Metabolic Confusion to Overcome Plateaus

To effectively use metabolic confusion to break through a weight loss plateau, it's essential to plan and track your calorie intake carefully. Here's how you can start:

1. **Calculate Your Caloric Needs**: Begin by determining your maintenance calories—the amount you need to consume to maintain your current weight. Numerous online calculators can help you find this number based on your age, gender, weight, height, and activity level.

2. **Plan Your High and Low-Calorie Days**: Once you know your maintenance calories, plan your week with a mix of high and low-calorie days. For example, you might consume 200-300 calories above your maintenance level on high days and 200-300 calories below on low days. Ensure you're still meeting your nutritional needs on low-calorie days.

3. **Monitor Your Progress and Adjust**: Keep a close eye on how your body responds. If you're not seeing the desired results, you may need to adjust your calorie targets. Remember, the key is to create enough of a variation to stimulate your metabolism without causing nutritional deficiencies or excessive calorie surpluses.

4. **Incorporate Exercise**: Exercise, particularly strength training, is a vital component of overcoming a weight loss plateau. It helps build muscle, which can increase your resting metabolic rate, making your metabolic confusion diet even more effective.

5. **Stay Hydrated and Prioritize Sleep**: Often overlooked, hydration and sleep play crucial roles in metabolism and weight loss. Ensure you're drinking enough water and getting adequate rest to support your body's fat-burning processes.

UNDERSTANDING BODY TYPES

Overview of Different Body Types

The Concept of Somatotypes

The theory of somatotypes was developed in the early 20th century by psychologist William Herbert Sheldon. He identified three primary body types based on a person's physical build and composition: ectomorph, mesomorph, and endomorph. It's important to note that very few people fit perfectly into one category; most of us are a blend, exhibiting characteristics of two or even all three types. Understanding these can be a powerful tool in crafting a lifestyle that harmonizes with our body's natural tendencies.

Ectomorphs: The Linear and Lanky

Ectomorphs are often described as the "linear" body type. They tend to have a slim, long, and lean physique, with smaller bone structures and less natural muscle mass compared to the other types. Ectomorphs might find it challenging to gain weight, both in terms of muscle and fat, due to their fast metabolism. This body type epitomizes the phrase "skinny genes," as they can eat substantial amounts without gaining much weight.

Key Characteristics:

- Slim and lean body
- Fast metabolism
- Difficulty gaining muscle and fat
- Narrow shoulders and hips

Optimal Strategies:

- **Nutrition:** Ectomorphs benefit from a higher intake of healthy carbohydrates and proteins to fuel their metabolism and support muscle growth. Frequent, nutrient-dense meals can help in gaining weight and building muscle.
- **Fitness:** Strength training with heavier weights and lower repetitions can be effective, along with adequate rest between workouts to promote muscle recovery and growth.

Mesomorphs: The Naturally Muscular

Mesomorphs are the "middle ground" body type, characterized by a naturally athletic physique with a well-defined musculature. They have a moderate to high bone density, a strong body, and an efficient metabolism that balances muscle gain and fat loss effectively. Mesomorphs are adaptable and can typically gain muscle and lose fat relatively easily compared to the other types.

Key Characteristics:

- Athletic and muscular build
- Efficient metabolism
- Balanced body composition
- Broad shoulders

Optimal Strategies:

- **Nutrition:** A balanced diet rich in proteins, carbohydrates, and fats supports the mesomorph's need for energy and muscle repair. Portion control and meal timing can help optimize body composition.

- **Fitness:** A combination of strength training and cardiovascular exercise suits mesomorphs well, allowing them to build muscle and maintain a lean physique.

Endomorphs: The Solid and Strong

Endomorphs possess a solid and often rounder physique, with a predisposition to store more fat. They have a wider bone structure, especially in the hips and waist, which contributes to their body's tendency to retain weight. Endomorphs may find it more challenging to lose fat, but they also have the advantage of gaining muscle relatively easily.

Key Characteristics:

- Solid and soft body
- Slower metabolism
- Tendency to gain fat and muscle
- Wide hips and shoulders

Optimal Strategies:

- **Nutrition:** A diet higher in protein and lower in carbohydrates, with an emphasis on whole, unprocessed foods, can help manage weight and support muscle maintenance and growth.
- **Fitness:** High-intensity interval training (HIIT) and strength training can be particularly effective for fat loss and muscle building. Consistency and intensity are key to overcoming the metabolic challenges.

Characteristics of Endomorph Body Type

When embarking on a journey to better health and fitness, understanding your body type is like being handed the map in a treasure hunt. It guides you through the maze of dieting advice, workout routines, and lifestyle changes towards the treasure of optimal health. For us endomorph ladies, this understanding is crucial. So, let's delve into the world of the endomorph body type, understanding its characteristics, its beauty, and how to navigate its challenges with grace and strategy.

The Essence of the Endomorph

Imagine the endomorph body as the Earth element—solid, grounded, and full of potential. Endomorphs are characterized by a fuller figure, with a tendency to store more fat, particularly around the midsection, hips, and thighs. Our bones are often short and thick, giving us a strong, sturdy appearance. This body type can be seen as the epitome of femininity, with soft, curvaceous lines that have been celebrated in art and culture throughout history.

However, the endomorph body type is not just about appearance. It comes with a unique set of metabolic characteristics. Our bodies are incredibly efficient at storing energy, which historically would have been a boon. In today's world of abundant food, however, this efficiency can feel more like a curse, making weight management a challenge.

The metabolism of an endomorph tends to be slower, which means we burn calories at a more leisurely pace compared to our ectomorph and mesomorph counterparts. This slow burn affects how we approach food and exercise. While it might seem unfair, it's simply a matter of understanding this metabolic melody and learning how to compose a lifestyle that harmonizes with it.

Strengths in the Shadows

Before we dive into the strategies for thriving as an endomorph, let's talk about the strengths. Yes, you heard that right—strengths. Our bodies are powerhouse machines when it comes to activities that require stamina and strength. We excel in sports and exercises that need sustained effort, from rowing to cycling to powerlifting. Our muscle fibers are built for endurance, and when properly trained, they shine. Moreover, the endomorph body is resilient. We have the capacity to handle heavy workout sessions, and with the right training, we can sculpt our muscles to be strong and defined. Our bodies respond well to resistance training, making it a key ally in our fitness journey.

Navigating the Challenges

Understanding the characteristics of the endomorph body type is the first step. The next step is navigating the challenges with wisdom and strategy. Here's how:

1. **Diet Wisdom:** Our bodies thrive on a well-balanced diet, rich in nutrients, and moderated in carbohydrates. Since our metabolism leans on the slower side, managing carb intake becomes crucial. Opting for complex carbohydrates, fiber-rich veggies, and lean proteins can help manage blood sugar levels and support weight management. It's about quality over quantity, choosing foods that nourish and satisfy without overburdening our metabolic system.

2. **The Magic of Movement:** Regular exercise is non-negotiable for us. But not just any exercise; a mix of cardiovascular workouts to boost heart health and burn fat, coupled with strength training to build muscle and enhance metabolism. Embrace activities you love, from dancing to swimming to weightlifting, ensuring consistency becomes a joy rather than a chore.

3. **Rest and Recharge:** Never underestimate the power of good sleep and stress management. Our bodies, sensitive to stress, can hold onto weight as a defense mechanism. Practices like yoga, meditation, and ensuring quality sleep can help mitigate stress, supporting overall health and weight management efforts.

4. **Hydration and Hormones:** Staying hydrated and managing hormonal balance are keys to unlocking our metabolic potential. Water aids in digestion and metabolism, while hormonal imbalances can sabotage our best efforts. Paying attention to how our bodies respond to different foods and activities can guide us in maintaining this delicate balance.

Challenges and Strategies for Endomorph Women

Our body type, characterized by a greater tendency to store fat, a wider frame, and a slower metabolism, presents unique challenges that can make traditional dieting and exercise advice seem ineffective, if not downright discouraging. But within these challenges lies the opportunity for profound growth and understanding. Let's explore these challenges together and, more importantly, uncover the strategies that can lead us to our wellness goals.

Understanding Our Unique Challenges

1. **Slower Metabolism:** Our bodies tend to have a slower metabolic rate, meaning we burn calories at a slower pace than our ectomorph or mesomorph counterparts. This can lead to weight gain or difficulty losing weight, even with a calorie-restricted diet.

2. **Predominance of Fat Storage:** Endomorphs are genetically predisposed to store fat more readily, particularly around the abdomen, hips, and thighs. This fat distribution pattern can be a source of frustration, especially when striving for weight loss.

3. **Insulin Sensitivity:** Many endomorphs experience a higher degree of insulin sensitivity, which can lead to increased fat storage when consuming a diet high in refined carbs and sugars.

4. **Difficulty Gaining Muscle:** While endomorphs can build muscle, the presence of higher fat levels can make it challenging to see muscle definition, leading to discouragement in strength training efforts.

Embracing Effective Strategies

While these challenges may seem daunting, the good news is that with the right strategies, endomorph women can achieve their health and fitness goals. Here's how:

1. Tailoring Your Nutrition:

- **Focus on Whole Foods:** Prioritize a diet rich in vegetables, fruits, lean proteins, and healthy fats. Whole foods are not only nutrient-dense but also provide the fiber needed to keep you full and support a healthy metabolism.

- **Control Carbohydrate Intake:** Given the tendency towards insulin sensitivity, moderating your carb intake, especially refined carbs, is crucial. Opt for complex carbohydrates like whole grains, legumes, and vegetables that provide a slow and steady release of energy.
- **Frequent, Balanced Meals:** Eating smaller, balanced meals more frequently throughout the day can help manage hunger and stabilize blood sugar levels, preventing overeating.

2. Optimizing Your Exercise Routine:

- **Incorporate Strength Training:** Muscle burns more calories at rest than fat, so building muscle is key for boosting metabolism. Focus on compound movements like squats, deadlifts, and bench presses that work multiple muscle groups.
- **Don't Skip Cardio:** While strength training should be a priority, incorporating cardio is also important for heart health and burning calories. Find a form of cardio you enjoy, whether it's brisk walking, cycling, or swimming.
- **Try High-Intensity Interval Training (HIIT):** HIIT can be particularly effective for endomorphs as it burns a lot of calories in a short amount of time and can increase metabolic rate even after the workout is done.

3. Managing Stress and Sleep:

- **Prioritize Sleep:** Quality sleep is essential for regulating hormones that control appetite and metabolism. Aim for 7-9 hours of sleep per night to support your weight loss efforts.
- **Manage Stress:** Chronic stress can lead to overeating and weight gain. Incorporate stress-reduction techniques like

meditation, yoga, or deep-breathing exercises into your daily routine.

4. Consistency and Patience:

- **Set Realistic Goals:** Achieving your health and fitness goals is a marathon, not a sprint. Set small, achievable goals that lead to long-term success.

- **Be Patient With Yourself:** Progress may be slower than you'd like, but remember, every step forward is a step in the right direction. Celebrate your victories, no matter how small.

METABOLIC CONFUSION DIET PHASES

High-Calorie Phase: Goals and Food List

The primary aim of the High-Calorie Phase is to fuel your metabolism into a higher gear. It's about providing your body with enough energy and nutrients to signal that it's okay to burn fat, rather than conserve it. Here are the key goals we're looking to achieve:

1. **Boost Metabolism**: By increasing calorie intake, we encourage the body to maintain a higher metabolic rate. This is crucial for breaking through weight loss plateaus.

2. **Muscle Growth and Repair**: Higher calorie days support muscle synthesis and repair, especially important if you're incorporating strength training into your routine.

3. **Psychological Relief**: Let's be honest, dieting can be tough. Having days where you can eat more freely helps to keep motivation high and prevents feelings of deprivation.

4. **Hormonal Balance**: Restrictive diets can sometimes lead to hormonal imbalances, affecting everything from your mood to your ability to lose weight. The High-Calorie Phase helps to reset and balance these crucial hormones.

The High-Calorie Food List

Navigating the High-Calorie Phase doesn't mean you can eat anything and everything. The focus is on nutrient-dense foods that provide your body with the right kind of energy. Let's break it down:

Proteins

High-quality protein is your ally in building and repairing muscle. During this phase, aim to include:

- **Lean Meats**: Chicken breast, turkey, and lean cuts of beef or pork.
- **Fish**: Salmon, tuna, and mackerel not only provide protein but also essential omega-3 fatty acids.
- **Plant-Based Proteins**: Quinoa, lentils, chickpeas, and black beans are great for those looking to reduce animal protein consumption.

Carbohydrates

Carbs are your body's primary energy source, especially during the High-Calorie Phase. Opt for complex carbohydrates that provide sustained energy:

- **Whole Grains**: Brown rice, quinoa, barley, and whole wheat products.
- **Starchy Vegetables**: Sweet potatoes, yams, and butternut squash.
- **Legumes**: Lentils, chickpeas, and beans also fall into this category, providing both protein and carbs.

Fats

Healthy fats are essential for hormone production and nutrient absorption:

- **Avocados**: Packed with monounsaturated fats and fiber.
- **Nuts and Seeds**: Almonds, walnuts, chia seeds, and flaxseeds offer healthy fats and protein.
- **Olive Oil**: A great source of healthy monounsaturated fats, perfect for cooking or dressings.

Fruits and Vegetables

Fruits and vegetables are packed with vitamins, minerals, and fiber, essential for overall health and digestion:

- **Fruits**: Berries, apples, bananas, and oranges. Don't shy away from fruits due to their natural sugars; they're packed with nutrients.
- **Vegetables**: Aim for a rainbow of colors to maximize nutrient intake. Spinach, kale, bell peppers, and carrots are all excellent choices.

Dairy or Dairy Alternatives

Calcium and vitamin D are important for bone health:

- **Greek Yogurt**: High in protein and probiotics.
- **Milk or Milk Alternatives**: Choose options that are fortified with calcium and vitamin D.

Tips for Success

1. **Balance Is Key**: Ensure each meal has a good balance of proteins, carbs, and fats. This not only supports your metabolic goals but also helps in keeping you satisfied.

2. **Portion Control**: High-calorie doesn't mean unlimited calories. Be mindful of portion sizes to avoid overeating.

3. **Listen to Your Body**: Use this phase to tune into your body's hunger and fullness signals. Eating more on some days shouldn't mean pushing past comfort.

4. **Stay Hydrated**: Sometimes thirst is mistaken for hunger. Keeping well-hydrated ensures that you're eating because you're truly hungry.

5. **Enjoy Your Food**: This phase is also about psychological relief, so choose foods that you genuinely enjoy and look forward to eating.

Low-Calorie Phase: Goals and Food List

The Low-Calorie Phase isn't just about cutting calories; it's about redefining our relationship with food and our bodies. The goals here are multi-layered, much like the stories we each carry within us.

1. **Encouraging Fat Loss:** At its core, this phase aims to gently nudge our bodies into using stored fat for energy. It's a kind, supportive whisper to our metabolism, encouraging it to explore the energy reserves we've lovingly stored over time.

2. **Maintaining Muscle Mass:** While the focus is on fat loss, we're also here to protect our muscle mass. It's about ensuring

that what we lose is fat, not the precious muscle that keeps us strong and our metabolisms humming.

3. **Nutritional Balance:** This phase is about nourishing our bodies, even with fewer calories. It's a testament to the fact that less can indeed be more when chosen with care and love.

4. **Metabolic Adaptation:** Here, we're teaching our bodies to adapt to different energy intakes without slowing down. It's a lesson in resilience and flexibility, qualities that mirror the strength within each of us.

The Food List

Embarking on the Low-Calorie Phase doesn't mean bidding farewell to flavorful, satisfying meals. On the contrary, it's about welcoming a variety of nutrient-rich foods that not only nourish but also delight. Here's a guide to the foods that will become your companions on this leg of the journey.

Proteins

Lean proteins are your allies, offering sustenance without excess calories. Think of them as the gentle, steady friends who support you without overwhelming.

- Chicken breast
- Turkey
- Fish, especially those rich in omega-3 like salmon and mackerel, but in moderation
- Legumes, including lentils and chickpeas
- Tofu and tempeh for plant-based strength
- Egg whites, a pure, simple source of protein

Carbohydrates

Carbs are not the enemy. In the Low-Calorie Phase, we choose them wisely, opting for those that provide energy and nutrients without spiking our blood sugar.

- Leafy greens, such as spinach, kale, and arugula, which are low in calories but rich in fiber and nutrients
- Cruciferous vegetables like broccoli and cauliflower, offering depth and texture to meals
- Berries, small but mighty sources of antioxidants and sweetness
- Whole grains, in moderation, such as quinoa and farro, for their satisfying substance and nutritional value

Fats

Healthy fats are crucial, even in a low-calorie phase. They're the richness in the tapestry of our diet, essential for absorbing vitamins and keeping our cells healthy.

- Avocado, in small portions, brings creaminess and heart-healthy fats
- Nuts and seeds, though calorie-dense, are powerful in tiny amounts
- Olive oil, a drizzle here and there for its monounsaturated fats and flavor

Vegetables and Fruits

Here, we dive into the garden of variety, choosing vegetables and fruits that fill us without weighing us down.

- Zucchini, eggplant, and other high-water content vegetables that offer volume and fiber

- Apples and oranges, portable snacks that combine fiber and sweetness
- Tomatoes and cucumbers, hydrating and refreshing

Beverages

Hydration is key, especially when managing calorie intake. Our choices here are simple but vital.

- Water, the essence of life, flavored with a slice of lemon or cucumber for a touch of elegance
- Herbal teas, a way to soothe and hydrate without calories
- Black coffee, for those who enjoy its robust wakefulness, minus the cream and sugar

Transitioning Between Phases

Before we delve into the transitions, let's quickly recap what we mean by high-calorie and low-calorie phases. In the high-calorie phase, you're consuming more calories than your body burns, providing it with ample energy and signaling it to ramp up its metabolic processes. This phase is not about indulging in unhealthy foods but about strategically increasing your intake of nutritious, calorie-dense foods.

Conversely, the low-calorie phase involves reducing your caloric intake below your body's energy needs. This encourages your body to turn to stored fat for energy, leading to weight loss. Like the high-calorie phase, the focus remains on nutritionally rich foods, ensuring your body gets the essential nutrients it needs to function optimally.

Planning Your Transition

Transitioning between these phases requires thoughtful planning. A sudden switch from high to low calories (or vice versa) can be a shock to your system, potentially causing cravings, fatigue, or even resistance to weight loss. Here's how to ease into transitions:

1. **Gradual Adjustment:** Instead of making an abrupt change, gradually adjust your caloric intake over a few days. For instance, if moving from a high-calorie to a low-calorie phase, slightly reduce your calorie intake each day over the course of 3-5 days. This helps your body and mind adjust without shock.

2. **Mindful Eating:** Pay close attention to how your body responds to changes in your diet. Are you feeling more energetic or perhaps a bit sluggish? Adjusting your caloric intake isn't just about numbers; it's about listening to your body and responding to its needs.

3. **Hydration and Sleep:** These two factors play a significant role in how effectively your body adapts to changes. Ensure you're well-hydrated and getting enough sleep, especially during transitions, to support your body's metabolic processes.

4. **Exercise Adjustment:** Your workout routine should align with your dietary phases. During high-calorie phases, focus on more intense workouts or strength training, taking advantage of the extra energy. As you transition to a low-calorie phase, consider reducing the intensity or volume of your workouts to match your lower energy intake.

Psychological Aspects of Transitioning

The psychological impact of transitioning between phases is as significant as the physical. It's common to experience a range of emotions, from excitement at the prospect of more varied meals in a high-calorie phase to apprehension about reducing calorie intake. Here's how to manage these psychological aspects:

1. **Set Realistic Expectations:** Understand that it's normal to feel hungry during the first few days of a low-calorie phase or unusually full at the start of a high-calorie phase. Setting realistic expectations can help you navigate these feelings without becoming discouraged.

2. **Stay Flexible:** Some days, you might find it harder to stick to your planned caloric intake. Instead of viewing this as a failure, see it as an opportunity to learn and adapt. Flexibility is key to a sustainable metabolic confusion approach.

3. **Support System:** Share your journey with friends, family, or a support group who understand and support your goals. Having someone to talk to can make the transitions easier and more enjoyable.

Nutritional Strategies for Smoother Transitions

Nutrition plays a pivotal role in how smoothly you can transition between phases. Here are some strategies to consider:

1. **Focus on Fiber:** During both phases, but especially when transitioning into a low-calorie phase, incorporate plenty of high-fiber foods. Fiber helps you feel fuller longer, making the reduction in calories less noticeable.

2. **Protein is Key:** Maintaining a high protein intake can help preserve muscle mass, especially important during the low-calorie phase. Protein also aids in satiety, helping you feel satisfied.

3. **Manage Carbohydrates:** In the high-calorie phase, prioritize complex carbohydrates (like whole grains and vegetables) for sustained energy. When transitioning to a low-calorie phase, you may want to slightly reduce your carbohydrate intake, especially from processed sources, to help manage your overall calorie reduction.

4. **Healthy Fats:** Don't shy away from healthy fats, even in a low-calorie phase. Fats like avocados, nuts, and olive oil can keep you feeling satisfied and support your body's nutritional needs.

FOODS TO EAT

Proteins

Protein is like that reliable friend who's always there to help you rebuild and recover. After a workout, when your muscles are like, "What just happened?!" protein steps in, whispering, "I got you." It goes to work repairing those tiny tears caused by exercising, helping your muscles come back stronger and ready for more.

But protein's role isn't just about recovery; it's also about growth. For us endomorph ladies, building lean muscle is like striking gold in our metabolic efficiency quest. More muscle means a higher resting metabolic rate, meaning you burn more calories even when you're not hitting the gym. It's like your body becomes a more efficient energy-burning fireplace, with protein logs keeping the fire roaring.

Now, not all proteins are created equal. Imagine walking into a boutique where every piece of clothing is tailored to make you look and feel fabulous. That's how you should approach selecting your proteins – choose quality sources that your body can use efficiently. Lean meats like chicken, turkey, and fish are fantastic, as they're like the haute couture of proteins, stylishly fitting into your diet while providing essential nutrients.

For my plant-based friends, fear not. Legumes, lentils, tofu, and tempeh are like the versatile basics in your wardrobe, pairing well with almost anything while offering a hefty protein punch. And let's not forget about quinoa and chia seeds, the accessories that complete the outfit, adding that extra flair of protein to your meals.

But how much protein do you need? Picture this: you're painting a masterpiece, and protein is your paint. Too little, and your canvas looks bare; too much, and it loses its charm. The right amount varies for each of us, depending on our lifestyle, weight, and fitness goals. A common starting point is aiming for about 1.2 to 2.0 grams of protein per kilogram of body weight, especially if you're active and looking to build muscle. It's like adjusting the brightness and contrast on a photo until it's just right – it requires a bit of tweaking to find your perfect protein setting.

Here's where the magic of metabolic confusion comes in. By varying your protein intake along with your calories, you can keep your metabolism guessing and your body thriving. On high-calorie days, amp up the protein with hearty dishes like grilled chicken salads or lentil stews. On lower-calorie days, lean into lighter fare, like smoothies boosted with plant-based protein powder or a delicate fish fillet with steamed veggies.

Food	Portion Size	Protein (g)	Calories	Fat (g)	Carbs (g)
Almonds	1 oz	6	164	14	6.1
Black beans	1 cup	15	227	1	41
Canned mackerel	100g	24	205	13.9	0
Canned sardines	100g	25	208	11	0

Casein protein powder	30g	24	120	1	3
Chia seeds	2 tbsp	4	138	8.7	12.3
Chicken breast	100g	31	165	3.6	0
Chickpeas	1 cup	14.5	269	4.2	45
Cottage cheese	1 cup	14	163	2.3	6.1
Edamame	100g	11	188	5	13.8
Eggs	1 large	6	78	5	0.6
Greek yogurt	1 cup	10	59	0.4	3.6
Hemp seeds	2 tbsp	9	166	14.6	2.6
Kidney beans	1 cup	13	225	0.9	40.4
Lean beef	100g	26	250	15	0
Lentils	1 cup	18	230	0.8	40
Parmesan cheese	100g	35	431	29	3.8
Pea protein powder	30g	21	120	1.5	2
Peanuts	1 oz	7	161	14	4.6
Pork tenderloin	100g	23	143	3.5	0

Quinoa	1 cup	8	222	3.6	39.4
Salmon	100g	25	208	13	0
Skim milk	1 cup	8	83	0.2	12
Soy milk	1 cup	8	80	4	4
Spirulina	2 tbsp	4	20	0.5	1.7
Swiss cheese	100g	25	380	27	1.5
Tempeh	100g	19	195	10.8	7.6
Tofu	100g	8	76	4.8	1.9
Tuna	100g	29	184	1.3	0
Turkey breast	100g	29	135	1.6	0
Walnuts	1 oz	4	185	18.5	3.9
Whey protein powder	30g	24	120	1	3
Feta cheese	100g	14	264	21	4
Mozzarella cheese	100g	28	280	17	3.1
Ricotta cheese	100g	11	174	10	3
Broccoli	1 cup	2.8	31	0.4	6
Spinach	1 cup	2.9	23	0.4	3.6
Asparagus	1 cup	2.2	20	0.2	3.9

Kale	1 cup	2.9	49	0.9	8.8
Brussels sprouts	1 cup	3.4	43	0.3	8.9
Turkey bacon	100g	20	89	5	1.1
Canadian bacon	100g	17	72	2.4	1.2
Venison	100g	26	158	7	0
Bison	100g	28	174	7.2	0
Cod	100g	18	105	0.7	0
Haddock	100g	20	95	0.7	0
Halibut	100g	22	111	2.3	0
Tilapia	100g	26	128	2.7	0
Soybeans	1 cup	17	188	8.9	14.3
Navy beans	1 cup	15	225	1.1	47.3
Pumpkin seeds	1 oz	7	158	13.5	1.7
Sunflower seeds	1 oz	5.5	164	14.4	6.5
Greek yogurt (non-fat)	1 cup	23	120	0.4	9
Flaxseeds	2 tbsp	3.8	110	8.8	6
Cashews	1 oz	5	157	12.3	9.2

Pistachios	1 oz	6	159	12.8	7.7
Mackerel	100g	24	205	13.9	0

Carbohydrates

Carbohydrates are the body's primary energy source, fueling everything from our brain function to our workouts. However, the key to harnessing their power without derailing our goals lies in choosing complex carbohydrates over their simple counterparts.

Complex carbohydrates are like the slow-burning logs in a fireplace, providing a steady, sustained release of energy. They're found in foods like whole grains, legumes, and vegetables, which are not only packed with energy but also rich in fiber, vitamins, and minerals. This fiber content is crucial, as it helps regulate our blood sugar levels, keeping us full longer and preventing the spikes and crashes associated with simple sugars.

Simple carbohydrates, on the other hand, are the quick-burning paper in our metaphorical fireplace. They ignite and burn out rapidly, leading to those all-too-familiar energy highs followed by lows. Found in processed foods, sugary snacks, and white bread, simple carbs offer little nutritional value and can sabotage our metabolic goals if not managed carefully.

Timing Is Everything

When it comes to carbohydrates, timing can be just as important as the type. Incorporating strategic carbohydrate timing into our metabolic confusion diet can enhance our metabolism, support our workout performance, and aid in recovery.

1. **Pre-Workout:** Consuming a moderate amount of complex carbohydrates about an hour before exercising can provide the sustained energy needed to power through a workout. Think of it as laying the groundwork for optimal performance, ensuring your body has the fuel it needs to excel.

2. **Post-Workout:** After a workout, your body is primed for recovery, making it the perfect time to introduce a mix of carbohydrates and protein. This is when simple carbohydrates can actually be beneficial, as they're quickly absorbed, helping to replenish glycogen stores and repair muscle when paired with protein. A fruit smoothie with a scoop of protein powder can be an ideal post-workout snack.

3. **Throughout the Day:** For the rest of the day, focus on complex carbohydrates, distributing them evenly across meals to maintain energy levels, support metabolic health, and prevent hunger pangs. Integrating these carbs with healthy fats and proteins can further stabilize blood sugar and satiety.

Food	Portion Size	Calories (kcal)	Carbs (g)	Fiber (g)	Sugars (g)	Protein (g)	Fat (g)
Acorn Squash	1 cup cubed	115	30	9	0	2	0.2
Adzuki Beans	1/2 cup	147	28.2	7.3	0	8.5	0.2
Arborio Rice	1 cup cooked	204	44	0.6	0	4.3	0.6
Barley Flakes	1 cup cooked	96	22	3	0	2	0.5
Basmati Rice	1 cup cooked	210	45	0.6	0.1	4.4	0.5
Black Quinoa	1 cup cooked	228	40	5	2	8	3.5
Black Rice	1 cup cooked	200	34	5	0	6	1.5
Black-eyed Peas	1/2 cup	99	17.7	5.6	2.3	6.7	0.4
Buckwheat Groats	1 cup cooked	155	33.5	4.5	0	5.7	1
Bulgur	1 cup cooked	151	33.8	8.2	0.2	5.6	0.4
Butternut Squash	1 cup cubed	82	22	6.6	4	1.8	0.2
Cannellini Beans	1/2 cup	100	18.5	6.3	0.6	7.3	0.4
Cassava	1 cup cubed	330	78.4	3.7	3.5	2.8	0.6

Chickpea Pasta	1 cup cooked	190	32	8	5	14	3.5
Couscous	1 cup cooked	176	36	2.2	0.2	5.9	0.3
Dates	1 cup	415	110	12.3	93	3.6	0.6
Dragon Fruit	1 cup	136	29	7	8	3	0
Ezekiel Bread	1 slice	80	15	3	0	4	0.5
Farro	1 cup cooked	200	37	7.5	1.5	7	1.5
Fava Beans	1/2 cup	94	16.7	4.3	1.2	6.1	0.4
Figs	1 cup	74	19.2	2.9	16.3	0.8	0.3
Freekeh	1 cup cooked	222	47.9	11.2	0	8.3	1.2
French Lentils	1/2 cup	115	20	8	2	9	0.4
Garbanzo Beans	1/2 cup	134	22.5	6.2	4	7.3	2.1
Great Northern Beans	1/2 cup	104	18.7	6.2	0.3	7.1	0.4
Green Banana	1 medium	105	27	3.1	14.4	1.3	0.4
Green Lentils	1/2 cup	114	20	7.8	1.8	9	0.4

Jasmine Rice	1 cup cooked	205	45	0.6	0.1	4.2	0.4
Jicama	1 cup sliced	46	11	6	2	0.9	0.1
Kamut	1 cup cooked	227	47.4	7.4	6.5	9.8	1.3
Kidney Beans	1/2 cup	113	20.1	7.3	0.3	7.7	0.5
Lentil Pasta	1 cup cooked	180	34	8	1	13	1.5
Lima Beans	1/2 cup	108	20	7	3	6.6	0.4
Millet	1 cup cooked	207	41	2.3	0.2	6.1	1.7
Mung Bean Noodles	1 cup cooked	190	47	0.3	0	0.1	0.1
Mung Beans	1/2 cup	106	19.2	7.6	0	7.0	0.4
Navy Beans	1/2 cup	127	23.7	9.6	0.4	7.5	0.6
Oat Bran	1 cup cooked	88	25	6	0.5	7	1.9
Parsnips	1 cup sliced	100	24	6.5	6.4	1.6	0.4
Pinto Beans	1/2 cup	122	22	7.7	0.2	7.2	0.6

Plantains	1 cup sliced	179	48	3.5	22	1.9	0.5
Polenta	1 cup cooked	98	23	2.5	0.2	2	0.5
Prunes	1 cup	418	111	12	66	3.8	0.7
Quinoa Flakes	1 cup	317	69.3	5.2	0	11.1	5.3
Raisins	1 cup	434	115	5.4	85.8	4.6	0.6
Red Lentils	1/2 cup	115	20	7.8	1.8	9	0.4
Red Quinoa	1 cup cooked	222	39	5	1.9	8.1	3.5
Rutabaga	1 cup cubed	52	12	3.2	6.2	1.5	0.2
Rye Flakes	1 cup cooked	100	23	5	0.5	4	1
Soba Noodles	1 cup cooked	113	24.4	1.3	0.1	5.8	0.1
Sorghum	1 cup cooked	214	44	3.3	0	5.4	1.6
Spelt	1 cup cooked	246	51	7.6	0.4	10.7	1.7
Sushi Rice	1 cup cooked	191	42	0.7	0	3.5	0.4
Taro	1 cup cubed	187	46.4	6.7	0.9	0.6	0.1
Tri-color Quinoa	1 cup cooked	220	39	5	1.5	8	3.5

Turnips	1 cup cubed	36	8.4	2.3	4.6	1.2	0.1
Wheat Bran	1/4 cup raw	30	18	12	0	4	1
Wild Rice	1 cup cooked	166	35	3	1	6.5	0.6

Fats

First things first, not all fats are created equal. There's been a significant shift in how we view fats in our diet, moving from a fat-phobic approach to understanding that fats—specifically, the healthy kinds—are vital to our health. Healthy fats are like the unsung heroes of our body's daily operations, supporting cell growth, protecting our organs, and providing us with essential fatty acids that our bodies can't produce on their own.

There are a few key players in the healthy fats lineup: monounsaturated and polyunsaturated fats, including the famous omega-3 and omega-6 fatty acids. You'll find these good guys in foods like avocados, nuts, seeds, and fish. They're the kind of fats that, when invited to the party, actually do your body good, helping to lower bad cholesterol levels, reduce inflammation, and even support brain health.

Now, let's talk about how these healthy fats fit into the metabolic confusion diet, especially for us endomorphs. Incorporating healthy fats into our diet can actually aid in weight management. Yes, you heard that right. When we include sources of healthy fats in our meals, they help us feel fuller longer, reducing the urge to snack on less healthy options. Plus, they're essential for absorbing vitamins A, D, E, and K, making sure we're getting the full benefit from our meals.

But how do we balance it all? It's all about moderation and making smart choices. Instead of reaching for a bag of chips, opt for a handful of almonds or a slice of avocado. When cooking, choose oils like olive or canola, known for their heart-healthy properties. And don't forget about fish – incorporating fatty fish like salmon into your diet a couple of times a week can boost your intake of omega-3s, supporting heart and brain health.

Food Item	Portion Size	Saturated Fat (g)	Monounsaturated Fat (g)	Polyunsaturated Fat (g)	Other Nutrients
Avocado	1/2 medium	2.1	9.8	1.8	Fiber: 6.7g
Almonds	1 oz (28g)	1.1	8.8	3.4	Protein: 6g
Chia Seeds	1 tbsp	0.9	0.6	7.0	Omega-3: 5g
Olive Oil	1 tbsp	2.0	10	1.5	Vitamin E: 1.9mg
Flaxseeds	1 tbsp	0.4	0.8	2.9	Omega-3: 2.3g
Walnuts	1 oz (28g)	1.7	2.5	13	Omega-3: 2.5g
Coconut Oil	1 tbsp	12	0.8	0.2	-
Dark Chocolat	1 oz (28g)	7.0	4.0	0.5	Iron: 3.3mg

e (70-85%)					
Salmon (wild)	3 oz	1.5	3.8	4.0	Omega-3: 2.6g
Egg (whole)	1 large	1.6	2.0	0.7	Protein: 6g
Peanut Butter (natural)	2 tbsp	3.3	7.7	4.4	Protein: 8g
Cashews	1 oz (28g)	2.2	6.7	2.2	Magnesium: 82mg
Macadamia Nuts	1 oz (28g)	3.4	16.7	0.4	Manganese: 1.2mg
Sesame Seeds	1 tbsp	0.6	1.7	2.0	Calcium: 88mg
Pumpkin Seeds	1 oz (28g)	2.5	4.0	6.0	Magnesium: 150mg
Sunflower Seeds	1 oz (28g)	1.5	2.7	9.2	Vitamin E: 5.6mg
Greek Yogurt (full-fat)	100g	3.3	1.3	0.1	Protein: 9g
Grass-fed Butter	1 tbsp	7.0	3.0	0.5	Vitamin A: 355IU
Hemp Seeds	1 tbsp	0.5	0.5	3.5	Omega-3: 1g
Sardines (canned in oil)	1 can (92g)	1.5	3.8	5.1	Omega-3: 2.2g

Mackerel (wild)	3 oz	3.9	6.3	5.2	Omega-3: 2.6g
Cod Liver Oil	1 tsp	1.0	2.0	1.0	Vitamin D: 450IU
Tahini	1 tbsp	1.1	3.1	3.5	Calcium: 64mg
Brazil Nuts	1 oz (28g)	4.5	7.0	6.8	Selenium: 544µg
Avocado Oil	1 tbsp	2.0	10	2.0	-
Ghee	1 tbsp	9.3	4.5	0.5	Vitamin A: 8% DV
Hazelnuts	1 oz (28g)	1.3	12.8	2.2	Vitamin E: 21% DV
Pistachios	1 oz (28g)	1.6	6.8	3.9	Vitamin B6: 0.4mg
Fatty Tuna (raw)	3 oz	1.0	1.5	1.5	Omega-3: 1.3g
Trout (wild)	3 oz	1.0	2.3	2.9	Omega-3: 1g
Anchovies (canned)	1 oz (28g)	1.0	1.2	1.4	Omega-3: 1.2g
Olives (black)	1 oz (28g)	1.0	5.0	0.8	Fiber: 3g
Coconut Milk	1/4 cup	10	0.5	0.2	Manganese: 0.4mg
Pecans	1 oz (28g)	1.8	11.6	6.1	Fiber: 2.7g

Pine Nuts	1 oz (28g)	1.4	5.3	9.7	Iron: 1.6mg
Full-fat Cheese	1 oz (28g)	6.0	2.6	0.3	Calcium: 204mg
Borage Oil	1 tsp	1.0	2.0	2.0	Omega-6: 2g
Krill Oil	1 tsp	0.5	1.0	2.5	Omega-3: 1g
Duck Fat	1 tbsp	4.5	6.3	1.5	-
Grass-fed Beef Tallow	1 tbsp	6.0	5.5	0.5	-
Lard	1 tbsp	5.0	5.8	1.4	Vitamin D: 2.8μg
Soy Nuts	1 oz (28g)	1.5	2.2	5.9	Protein: 11g
Black Seed Oil	1 tsp	0.4	1.6	2.6	Thymoquinone: -
Camelina Oil	1 tbsp	1.0	3.6	9.0	Omega-3: 3.9g
Cottage Cheese (full-fat)	1/2 cup	3.2	1.4	0.1	Protein: 14g
Roasted Turkey (skin on)	3 oz	2.0	2.4	1.8	Protein: 24g
Grass-fed Lamb	3 oz	4.5	4.0	0.8	Protein: 23g

Clarified Butter (Ghee)	1 tbsp	9.3	4.5	0.5	Vitamin A: 8% DV

Vegetables and Fruits

First off, let's talk about why these natural goodies are so crucial. Vegetables and fruits are rich in vitamins, minerals, fiber, and antioxidants—each element playing a unique role in our health. The fiber keeps our digestive system running smoothly, ensuring we feel fuller for longer, which is essential on lower-calorie days. The vitamins and minerals keep our energy levels up and our bodies functioning optimally, while antioxidants fight off the free radicals that can lead to disease. But there's more to it than just their nutritional profile.

In the context of metabolic confusion, vegetables and fruits do something pretty remarkable. Their variety and versatility make them perfect for both high-calorie and low-calorie days. On high-calorie days, they can be part of nutrient-dense, satisfying meals, contributing to the overall caloric intake without the downside of processed foods. On low-calorie days, their low energy density means you can eat more of them—helping you feel full and satisfied without overdoing it on calories.

But here's the kicker: the vast array of fruits and vegetables available to us means we can constantly introduce new flavors and textures into our diet, keeping our meals interesting and our metabolism guessing. Think spicy peppers one day, sweet berries the next. Crunchy carrots followed by juicy tomatoes. This diversity isn't just good for our taste buds; it's a key player in the metabolic confusion game, helping to prevent dietary boredom and the dreaded weight loss plateau.

So, how do we make these heroes the star of our metabolic confusion journey? Variety and creativity are your best friends here. Aim to fill half your plate with vegetables at every meal, and include fruit as a regular part of your snacks or desserts. Explore different cooking methods—grilling, roasting, steaming—to bring out new flavors and textures. And don't be afraid to experiment with new, exotic fruits and vegetables that you've never tried before. Each new taste is an opportunity to engage your metabolism further.

Food	Portion Size	Calories (kcal)	Carbohydrates (g)	Protein (g)	Fat (g)	Fiber (g)
Almonds	1 oz	164	6.11	6	14.36	3.5
Apples	1 medium	95	25	0.5	0.3	4
Artichoke	1 medium	60	13.45	4.19	0.19	6.9
Arugula	1 cup	5	0.73	0.52	0.13	0.3
Asparagus	1 cup	27	5.2	2.95	0.16	2.8
Aubergine	1 cup	35	8.64	0.82	0.23	2.5
Avocado	1/4 medium	80	4	1	7	3
Bananas	1 medium	105	27	1.3	0.3	3.1
Beet Greens	1 cup	8	1.65	0.84	0.07	1.4
Beetroot	1 cup	58	13	2.2	0.2	3.8
Bell peppers	1 medium	24	5.5	1	0.2	1.5
Blackberries	1 cup	62	13.84	2	0.71	7.6
Blueberries	1 cup	84	21.45	1.1	0.49	3.6

Bok Choy	1 cup	9	1.5	1.05	0.14	0.7
Broccoli	1 cup	31	6	2.5	0.3	2.4
Brussels sprouts	1 cup	38	8	3	0.3	3.3
Butternut Squash	1 cup	63	16.37	1.4	0.14	2.8
Cabbage	1 cup	22	5.16	1.1	0.1	2.2
Cantaloupe	1 cup	53	13.67	1.31	0.3	1.4
Carrots	1 medium	25	5.84	0.57	0.15	1.7
Cauliflower	1 cup	25	5.3	2	0.1	2.5
Celery	1 cup	16	3.5	0.7	0.17	1.6
Chard	1 cup	7	1.35	0.65	0.07	0.6
Cherries	1 cup	87	22	1.5	0.3	3
Collard Greens	1 cup	11	2	1	0.15	1.3
Cranberries	1 cup	46	12.2	0.4	0.13	4.6
Cress	1 cup	4	0.85	0.31	0.06	0.1
Cucumbers	1 cup	16	3.89	0.8	0.2	0.5
Dandelion Greens	1 cup	25	5.1	1.5	0.4	1.9
Eggplant	1 cup	35	8.64	0.82	0.23	2.5
Endive	1 cup	8	1.77	0.64	0.1	1.6
Fennel	1 cup	27	6.34	1.08	0.17	2.7
Fig	1 medium	37	9.59	0.38	0.15	1.4
Garlic	1 clove	4	1	0.2	0	0.1
Ginger	1 tbsp	5	1.07	0.11	0.05	0.1
Grapefruit	1/2 medium	52	13.11	0.95	0.17	2
Grapes	1 cup	62	16	0.6	0.3	0.9

Green Beans	1 cup	31	7	1.8	0.22	3.4
Guava	1 cup	112	23.63	4.2	1.6	8.9
Honeydew Melon	1 cup	64	16	0.9	0.2	1.4
Jicama	1 cup	46	10.58	0.86	0.11	5.8
Kale	1 cup	33	6	2.9	0.6	1.3
Kiwi	1 medium	42	10.12	0.79	0.36	2.1
Kohlrabi	1 cup	36	8.37	2.26	0.1	4.9
Leeks	1 cup	54	12.59	1.34	0.34	1.6
Lemon	1 medium	17	5.41	0.64	0.17	1.6
Lettuce (Romaine)	1 cup	8	1.55	0.58	0.14	1
Lime	1 medium	20	7.06	0.47	0.13	1.9
Lychee	1 cup	125	31.4	1.58	0.83	2.5
Mache	1 cup	7	1	0.3	0.1	0.1
Mango	1 cup	99	24.7	1.4	0.6	2.6
Mushrooms	1 cup	15	2.3	2.2	0.2	0.7
Mustard Greens	1 cup	15	2.6	1.6	0.2	1.8
Nectarine	1 medium	63	15	1.5	0.4	2.4
Okra	1 cup	33	7.45	2	0.19	3.2
Onions	1 cup	64	14.94	1.76	0.16	2.7
Oranges	1 medium	62	15.39	1.23	0.16	3.1
Papaya	1 cup	62	16	0.7	0.4	2.5
Parsley	1 cup	22	3.8	1.78	0.47	2
Passion Fruit	1 fruit	17	4.02	0.4	0.13	1.9
Peaches	1 medium	58	14	1	0.4	2

Pears	1 medium	102	27.52	0.64	0.21	5.5
Peas	1 cup	117	21	7.9	0.6	7.4
Persimmon	1 medium	118	31.2	1	0.3	6
Pineapple	1 cup	82	21.65	0.89	0.2	2.3
Pomegranate	1/2 cup	72	16.3	1.5	1	3.5
Pumpkin	1 cup	30	8	1.2	0.1	0.6
Quinoa	1/4 cup	56	10	2	0.9	1.2
Radicchio	1 cup	9	1.8	0.6	0.1	0.9
Radishes	1 cup	19	4	0.8	0.1	1.9
Raspberries	1 cup	64	14.69	1.48	0.8	8
Rutabaga	1 cup	52	12	1.5	0.2	3.2
Snap Peas	1 cup	41	7.55	2.8	0.2	2.6
Spinach	1 cup	7	1.09	0.86	0.12	0.7
Spinach (cooked)	1 cup	41	6.75	5.35	0.47	4.32
Squash (summer)	1 cup	18	3.79	1.37	0.2	1.2
Squash (winter)	1 cup	76	19.85	1.82	0.71	5.74
Starfruit	1 fruit	28	6.73	1	0.27	2.8
Strawberries	1 cup	47	11	1	0.4	3
Sweet corn	1 cup	132	29.29	4.96	1.8	4.6
Sweet potatoes	1 medium	103	23.61	2.3	0.17	3.8
Tangerines	1 medium	47	11.7	0.7	0.3	1.6
Taro	1 cup	187	46.4	0.52	0.11	6.7
Tomatoes	1 medium	22	4.82	1.08	0.25	1.5

Turnips	1 cup	36	8.36	1.17	0.13	2.3
Ugli Fruit	1 fruit	90	22.5	1	0.3	2.5
Water Spinach	1 cup	11	2.01	1.03	0.12	1.2
Watercress	1 cup	4	0.4	0.8	0	0.2
Watermelon	1 cup	46	11.48	0.93	0.23	0.6
Yam	1 cup	177	41.82	2.3	0.26	6.1
Zucchini	1 cup	19	3.88	1.5	0.35	1
Zucchini Flowers	1 cup	5	0.78	0.41	0.06	0.3

Beverages

First things first, water is the cornerstone of any dietary strategy, including metabolic confusion. It's like the unsung hero that supports every bodily function, including our metabolism. Drinking adequate water can help maintain optimal metabolic rates, facilitating better energy use and fat burning. Moreover, water is a master of disguise, often quenching thirsts that our bodies might mistakenly interpret as hunger. By staying well-hydrated, we not only support our metabolism but also avoid unnecessary snacking, which is crucial for the low-calorie phases of metabolic confusion.

Coffee and tea, the darlings of the beverage world, come next with their complex characters. Both are celebrated for their antioxidant properties and, when consumed in moderation, can offer a metabolic boost thanks to caffeine. Caffeine stimulates the central nervous system, raising metabolism slightly and increasing fat burning. This makes your morning brew a valuable player in the metabolic confusion game, especially if you enjoy it black or with minimal additives. However, the key is moderation. Overdoing it can lead to dehydration or sleep disturbances, which might sabotage your metabolic efforts.

Smoothies and protein shakes represent a fantastic opportunity to align your beverage choices with the goals of metabolic confusion. On high-calorie days, they can be rich, nutrient-packed meals in a glass, providing an excellent balance of protein, healthy fats, and carbohydrates. On low-calorie days, a lighter version can serve as a satisfying snack or meal replacement that keeps your metabolism engaged without overdoing the calorie intake. The trick is to focus on whole, nutrient-dense ingredients like fruits, vegetables, and quality protein sources, steering clear of added sugars and high-calorie additives.

While exploring the landscape of beneficial beverages, it's crucial to shine a light on the ones best avoided or consumed sparingly: sugary sodas and processed juices. These are the trojan horses of the beverage world, often packed with added sugars and empty calories that can disrupt your metabolic confusion strategy. They spike your blood sugar and insulin levels, encouraging fat storage rather than burning. For someone navigating the metabolic confusion diet, replacing these with water, herbal teas, or homemade, no-sugar-added juices can make a significant difference.

Lastly, alcohol deserves a mention. While an occasional glass of wine or a light beer might not derail your efforts, regular or heavy consumption can. Alcohol provides empty calories, slows down metabolism, and can affect your judgment, leading to poorer food choices. Enjoying it in moderation or saving it for special occasions is a wise strategy within the metabolic confusion framework.

Beverage Type	Portion Size	Notes
Green Tea	1 cup (240ml)	Zero-calorie, metabolism-boosting
Black Coffee	1 cup (240ml)	Zero-calorie, can enhance fat burning
Almond Milk, unsweetened	1 cup (240ml)	Low in calories, dairy-free
Coconut Water	1 cup (240ml)	Hydrating, contains electrolytes
Kombucha (low-sugar)	1 cup (240ml)	Probiotic-rich, supports gut health
Whey Protein Shake	1 scoop in water	High in protein, supports muscle maintenance
Vegetable Juice, low sodium	1 cup (240ml)	Nutrient-dense, low in calories
Herbal Tea (unsweetened)	1 cup (240ml)	Variety of options for zero-calorie hydration
Sparkling Water	1 cup (240ml)	Zero-calorie, can aid in feeling full
Skim Milk	1 cup (240ml)	High in protein and calcium

Lemon & Mint Infused Water	1 cup (240ml)	Refreshing, aids digestion
Cucumber Infused Water	1 cup (240ml)	Low-calorie, hydrating
Chamomile Tea	1 cup (240ml)	Calming, zero-calorie
Peppermint Tea	1 cup (240ml)	Aids digestion, zero-calorie
Ginger Tea	1 cup (240ml)	May help with metabolism, zero-calorie
Berry Infused Water	1 cup (240ml)	Antioxidant-rich, low-calorie
Low-Calorie Vegetable Broth	1 cup (240ml)	Satisfying, can be nutrient-dense
Apple Cider Vinegar Drink	1 tbsp in water	May aid in weight management
Beet Juice	1 cup (240ml)	High in nutrients, supports stamina
Carrot Juice	1 cup (240ml)	Rich in beta-carotene, supports eye health
Tomato Juice, low sodium	1 cup (240ml)	Rich in lycopene, heart-healthy
Matcha Green Tea	1 cup (240ml)	High in antioxidants, metabolism-boosting
Rooibos Tea	1 cup (240ml)	Caffeine-free, rich in antioxidants

Hibiscus Tea	1 cup (240ml)	May help lower blood pressure, zero-calorie
Aloe Vera Juice	1 cup (240ml)	May support digestion, low-calorie
Celery Juice	1 cup (240ml)	Low-calorie, hydrating
Turmeric Tea (Golden Milk)	1 cup (240ml)	Anti-inflammatory properties
Bone Broth	1 cup (240ml)	Nutrient-dense, supports gut health
Pomegranate Juice	1 cup (240ml)	High in antioxidants, supports heart health
Watermelon Juice	1 cup (240ml)	Hydrating, low in calories
Cashew Milk, unsweetened	1 cup (240ml)	Dairy-free, low in calories
Rice Milk, unsweetened	1 cup (240ml)	Dairy-free, good for those allergic to nuts/soy
Oat Milk, unsweetened	1 cup (240ml)	Low in fat, dairy-free
Flaxseed Milk, unsweetened	1 cup (240ml)	High in omega-3 fatty acids, dairy-free
Hemp Milk, unsweetened	1 cup (240ml)	Contains omega-3 and omega-6, dairy-free
Ginger Lemon Hot Water	1 cup (240ml)	Aids digestion, immune-boosting

Dandelion Tea	1 cup (240ml)	May support liver health, zero-calorie
Licorice Tea	1 cup (240ml)	May soothe stomach, zero-calorie
Fennel Tea	1 cup (240ml)	Supports digestion, zero-calorie
Spearmint Tea	1 cup (240ml)	May improve hormone balance, zero-calorie
Cinnamon Tea	1 cup (240ml)	May help regulate blood sugar, zero-calorie
Seltzer Water with a Splash of Lime	1 cup (240ml)	Refreshing, zero-calorie
Cold Brew Coffee	1 cup (240ml)	Lower acidity than regular coffee, zero-calorie
Protein Infused Water	1 cup (240ml)	Supports muscle maintenance, low-calorie
Electrolyte Infused Water	1 cup (240ml)	Supports hydration, low-calorie
Unsweetened Soy Milk	1 cup (240ml)	High in protein, dairy-free
Miso Soup	1 cup (240ml)	Probiotic-rich, supports gut health
Sauerkraut Juice	1 cup (240ml)	Probiotic-rich, may aid digestion
Tart Cherry Juice	1 cup (240ml)	May aid muscle recovery, high in antioxidants

FOODS TO AVOID

Sugary and Processed Foods

Sugary foods, with their quick bursts of energy and dopamine, can be incredibly tempting. From the morning latte swirled with flavored syrup to the comfort of a chocolate bar after a long day, sugar has a way of sneaking into our daily routines. However, the immediate pleasure comes with a cost. These foods cause a rapid spike in blood sugar levels followed by an inevitable crash, leading to a cycle of cravings and energy dips. For those practicing metabolic confusion, the goal is to stabilize energy and blood sugar levels to support a more efficient metabolism. Consuming high amounts of sugar disrupts this balance, making it harder to shift between high and low-calorie phases effectively.

Processed foods often come packaged with convenience, long shelf life, and, unfortunately, a cocktail of additives, preservatives, and refined ingredients. While not all processed foods are detrimental— think canned beans or frozen vegetables—the majority offer little nutritional value and are high in calories, sodium, and unhealthy fats. These foods can dull our palate, making whole, nutrient-rich foods less appealing, and encourage overeating. In the context of metabolic confusion, where nutrient density and variety are key, processed foods can become roadblocks to achieving metabolic flexibility and health goals.

Food	Portion Size	Calories (kcal)	Carbs (g)	Sugar (g)	Fat (g)	Protein (g)
Soda	1 can (355ml)	150	39	39	0	0
Candy Bars	1 bar (50g)	250	33	28	14	3
Ice Cream	1/2 cup (105g)	137	16	14	7	2
Doughnuts	1 medium (4 oz)	255	31	15	15	4
Potato Chips	1 oz (28g)	155	14	1.2	10	2
White Bread	1 slice (25g)	67	13	2	1	2
Fast Food Burgers	1 medium burger	520	47	9	26	28
Fried Chicken	1 piece	320	8	0	24	14
French Fries	1 medium serving	365	48	0.4	17	4
Chocolate Cake	1 slice (64g)	249	35	24	12	3
Cookies	1 cookie (10g)	50	8	4	2	0.6
Muffins	1 medium (113g)	375	53	24	17	5
Sugary Cereals	1 cup (30g)	120	27	12	1	2

Fruit Yogurts	1 cup (245g)	230	42	39	3	11
Flavored Coffee Drinks	16 oz (473ml)	250	33	24	6	12
Energy Drinks	1 can (250ml)	110	28	27	0	0
Processed Meats (e.g., sausages)	2 oz (56g)	190	2	0	17	7
Canned Soup (high sodium)	1 cup (240ml)	150	20	6	5	4
White Pasta	1 cup cooked	220	43	2	1	8
White Rice	1 cup cooked	205	45	0	0.4	4.3
Bagels	1 medium (3 oz)	190	37	6	1	6
Croissants	1 large (67g)	272	30	6	14	5
Pancakes with Syrup	2 pancakes	520	97	12	12	8
BBQ Sauce	2 tbsp (30ml)	60	14	10	0	0
Ketchup	1 tbsp (17g)	20	5	4	0	0
Margarine	1 tbsp (14g)	100	0	0	11	0
Instant Noodles	1 package (85g)	380	51	2	14	9

Frozen Meals	1 meal (8 oz)	370	42	5	14	11
Granola Bars	1 bar (40g)	200	24	12	5	9
Pudding	1/2 cup (113g)	160	26	19	4	3.5
Fruit Snacks	1 package (23g)	80	19	11	0	0
Sports Drinks	1 bottle (591ml)	150	34	30	0	0
Sweetened Condensed Milk	1 oz (28g)	123	21	21	3	3
Canned Fruit in Syrup	1/2 cup (122g)	100	26	23	0	0
Cheese Puffs	1 oz (28g)	160	15	1	10	2
Syrupy Canned Vegetables	1/2 cup (121g)	90	22	14	0.5	0.2
Boxed Macaroni & Cheese	1 cup prepared	350	47	9	10	12
Store-bought Pie	1 slice (1/8 pie)	300	40	18	14	4
Cream Cheese Frosting	2 tbsp (35g)	140	18	16	0.5	7
Sweetened Iced Tea	1 cup (240ml)	90	22	22	0	0
Chocolate Syrup	2 tbsp (30ml)	100	24	20	0.5	1
Caramel Sauce	2 tbsp (30ml)	103	17	15	2.3	0

Hot Dogs	1 hot dog	150	2	0	14	5
Bologna	1 slice (28g)	90	1	0	7	8
Breakfast Cereals (sugary)	1 cup (30g)	110	26	12	1	0.5
Flavored Gelatin	1/2 cup (120g)	80	19	19	2	0
Packaged Cookies	4 cookies (28g)	140	20	10	2	6
Canned Baked Beans (sweetened)	1/2 cup (130g)	120	27	12	5	0.5
Milk Chocolate	1 oz (28g)	150	17	15	2	9
Flavored Milk	1 cup (240ml)	160	25	24	8	2.5
White Bagels	1 large (100g)	250	50	6	1.5	10
Cereal Bars	1 bar (45g)	190	25	15	6	2
Packaged Cupcakes	1 cupcake (53g)	220	29	24	10	2
Fruit Cocktail in Heavy Syrup	1/2 cup (122g)	110	28	23	0	0
Sweetened Applesauce	1 cup (246g)	200	50	36	0.2	0.4
Cheese Flavored Snacks	1 oz (28g)	160	14	2	10	2

Regular Soft Drinks	12 oz (355 ml)	140	39	39	0	0
Chocolate Covered Nuts	1 oz (28g)	160	15	13	10	3
Flavored Potato Chips	1 oz (28g)	160	15	1	10	2
Processed Cheese Slices	1 slice (21g)	70	1	0	6	4
Instant Mashed Potatoes	1 cup prepared	210	37	2	9	4
Canned Chili with Beans	1 cup (247g)	287	30	5	14	17
Boxed Cake Mix	1/10 package	280	53	35	3.5	3
Frozen Pizza	1/4 pizza	320	35	5	14	15
Microwave Popcorn	1 bag (100g)	535	58	0	30	9
Fruit Flavored Candy	10 pieces (40g)	150	37	30	0	0
Canned Pasta in Tomato Sauce	1 cup (260g)	200	34	12	2	6
Frozen Breakfast Sandwiches	1 sandwich	300	30	2	16	12
Store-Bought Frosting	2 tbsp (35g)	140	20	18	6	0
Flavored Water	1 bottle (500ml)	120	30	30	0	0
Sweetened Dried Fruits	1/4 cup (40g)	150	37	31	0	1

High-Fructose Corn Syrup	2 tbsp (30ml)	120	31	31	0	0
Pre-packaged Salads with Dressing	1 package (300g)	400	25	7	29	12
Sugar-Sweetened Iced Coffee	16 oz (473ml)	200	37	35	2.5	2
Flavored Creamers	1 tbsp (15ml)	35	5	5	1.5	0
Pre-made Pie Crusts	1/8 crust	100	10	2	7	1
Sugar-Sweetened Gelatin	1/2 cup (120g)	80	19	19	0	2
Canned Frosting	2 tbsp (33g)	140	21	18	5	0
Pre-sliced Fruit Loaf	1 slice (50g)	180	30	16	6	3
Flavored Rice Mixes	1 cup prepared	210	44	1	0.5	5
Instant Oatmeal Packets	1 packet (50g)	190	36	12	2.5	4
Flavored Tofu	1/2 cup (124g)	70	2	1	4	8
Pre-packaged Smoothies	8 oz (240ml)	200	37	32	1	3
Sugar-Sweetened Almond Milk	1 cup (240ml)	90	16	15	2.5	1
Flavored Syrups	2 tbsp (30ml)	100	26	20	0	0
Pre-made Cookie Dough	2 tbsp (28g)	120	16	10	6	1

Sugar-Sweetened Yogurt	1 cup (245g)	200	35	28	2	10
Flavored Popcorn	2 cups (16g)	90	10	6	5	2
Canned Condensed Soup	1 cup (240ml)	180	22	3	9	7
Boxed Brownie Mix	1/16 package	150	23	15	7	2
Flavored Cottage Cheese	1/2 cup (113g)	110	10	8	2.5	12
Pre-made Sushi Rolls	1 roll (200g)	300	60	10	2	6
Flavored Protein Bars	1 bar (60g)	220	24	18	9	20
Sugar-Sweetened Chewing Gum	1 piece (2.7g)	10	2	2	0	0
Flavored Non-Dairy Creamer	1 tbsp (15ml)	35	5	5	1.5	0
Pre-made Pasta Sauce	1/2 cup (128g)	90	13	9	3	2
Flavored Instant Tea	1 packet (23g)	90	22	22	0	0
Sugar-Sweetened Breakfast Pastries	1 pastry (50g)	200	25	15	10	3
Flavored Microwave Meals	1 meal (250g)	300	40	5	11	14
Pre-made Salad Dressing	2 tbsp (30ml)	140	2	1	15	0

High-Glycemic Carbohydrates

Before we dive deep, a quick refresher on the glycemic index (GI) is in order. The GI is a scale that ranks carbohydrates on a scale from 0 to 100, based on how quickly and how much they raise blood sugar levels after eating. Foods with a high GI are digested and absorbed rapidly, leading to a spike in blood sugar levels. This spike is the crux of the matter when we discuss HGCs.

High-glycemic carbohydrates, found in foods like white bread, most white rices, certain breakfast cereals, and sugary snacks, can provide a rapid energy boost. This makes them potentially useful in specific contexts, such as a quick pre-workout snack to provide immediate energy. However, the surge in blood sugar is often followed by a swift crash, leading to hunger pangs, cravings, and a potential derailment of dietary goals. This cycle of spike-and-crash can be particularly challenging for individuals following a metabolic confusion diet, aiming for a balanced and sustainable approach to weight management.

Incorporating HGCs into a metabolic confusion diet requires a strategic approach. On high-calorie days, when your diet allows for more carbohydrates, there might be a small window for including HGCs, especially around workout times when your body can use the quick energy release. However, the key lies in moderation and timing, ensuring that these high-glycemic carbs are consumed in a way that supports, rather than hinders, your metabolic goals.

One of the critical concerns with regular consumption of HGCs is their impact on insulin sensitivity. Over time, repeated blood sugar spikes can lead to increased insulin levels, contributing to insulin resistance. For individuals focusing on metabolic confusion and overall health, maintaining insulin sensitivity is paramount. It not only supports weight management but also helps in preventing chronic conditions like type 2 diabetes.

So, how do we navigate the inclusion of carbohydrates in a diet focused on metabolic confusion? The answer lies in opting for low to moderate glycemic index foods for the majority of your carb intake. Foods like sweet potatoes, quinoa, legumes, and most fruits offer a more gradual release of energy, keeping blood sugar levels stable and supporting sustained energy throughout the day.

However, it's not about entirely demonizing HGCs. Instead, it's about understanding their effects and strategically incorporating them into your diet in a way that aligns with your metabolic confusion plan. This might mean enjoying a slice of white bread or a serving of white rice post-exercise on a high-calorie day, when your body's immediate energy needs can utilize the quick sugar release effectively.

Food	Portion Size	Calories (kcal)	Carbs (g)	Fiber (g)	Sugars (g)	Protein (g)	Fat (g)
White Bread	1 slice (28g)	79	15	0.8	1.4	2.7	1
White Rice	1 cup cooked	204	44	0.6	0.1	4.2	0.4
Corn Flakes	1 cup (28g)	101	24	0.9	2	1.9	0.2
Pretzels	1 oz (28g)	108	22.5	0.9	0.9	2.6	0.8
Rice Cakes	1 cake (9g)	35	7.3	0.4	0.1	0.7	0.3
Instant Oatmeal	1 packet (28g)	100	19	3	3	4	2
Baked Potato	1 medium (173g)	161	37	3.8	1.7	4.3	0.2
Watermelon	1 cup diced	46	11.5	0.6	9.4	0.9	0.2
Pineapple	1 cup chunks	82	21.6	2.3	16	0.9	0.2
Banana	1 medium	105	27	3.1	14.4	1.3	0.4
Doughnuts	1 medium (64g)	255	31	1	15	3.6	15
Soda	1 can (355ml)	140	39	0	39	0	0
Candy Bars	1 bar (60g)	280	35	1	30	3	14
French Fries	1 medium serving	365	48	4.4	0.4	4	17

White Pasta	1 cup cooked	220	43	2.5	1.3	8	1.3
Bagels	1 medium (105g)	289	56	2	6	11	1.5
Croissants	1 large (67g)	272	30	2	6	5	14
White Baguette	1/4 baguette (57g)	145	29	1	0.8	5	0.6
Popcorn (buttered)	1 cup	58	6	1	0.1	1	3.3
Honey	1 tbsp (21g)	64	17	0	17	0.1	0
Maple Syrup	1 tbsp (20g)	52	13.4	0	12.1	0	0
White Sugar	1 tbsp (12g)	48	12.6	0	12.6	0	0
Fruit Yogurt (low-fat)	1 cup (245g)	155	33	0	31	5.3	1.5
Sports Drinks	1 bottle (500ml)	125	32	0	21	0	0
Breakfast Cereals (sweetened)	1 cup (30g)	112	26	0.7	12	1.7	0.2
Muffins (commercial)	1 medium (113g)	375	53	1.5	24	5	17
Ice Cream	1/2 cup (66g)	137	16	0.5	14	2.3	7
Fruit Cocktail (canned)	1 cup	109	28.2	1.8	27.2	0.6	0.2
Puffed Rice Cereal	1 cup (14g)	56	13	0	0.2	1	0.1

Rice Syrup	1 tbsp (20g)	55	14	0	8	0	0
Instant Mashed Potatoes	1 cup prepared	210	48	2	2	4	1
Rice Milk	1 cup (240ml)	113	22	0	10	0.7	2.3
Cornbread	1 piece (60g)	198	33	2.5	9	4.7	5.4
Graham Crackers	1 piece (14g)	59	11	0.5	4	1	1.4
Fruit Roll-Ups	1 roll (14g)	50	12	0	7	0	0.5
Waffles (frozen)	1 waffle (35g)	102	17	1	2	2.5	2.5
Pancake Syrup	1 tbsp (20g)	52	13.4	0	12.1	0	0
Gelatin Desserts	1/2 cup (120g)	80	19	0	18	2	0
Tapioca	1 cup cooked	544	135	1.5	5	0.3	0.1
Macaroni and Cheese (boxed)	1 cup prepared	350	47	2	6	10	15
Potato Chips	1 oz (28g)	152	14	1	0.1	2	10
Snack Cakes	1 cake (42g)	157	27	0.5	18	1	5
Candy (gummy)	1 oz (28g)	99	22	0	14	2	0
Dried Fruit	1/4 cup	100	25	2	18	1	0.2
Flavored Gelatin	1 cup prepared	80	19	0	18	2	0
Sweetened Condensed Milk	1 tbsp (20g)	61	10	0	10	1.5	1.5

Marshmallows	1 cup mini	159	41	0	29	1	0
Shortbread Cookies	4 cookies (40g)	210	25	0.5	6	2	11
Milk Chocolate	1 oz (28g)	152	17	1	15	2.2	8.5
Corn Syrup	1 tbsp (20g)	57	15.5	0	15.5	0	0
Soda Crackers	5 crackers (15g)	70	12	0.5	0	1	1.5
Vanilla Wafers	5 wafers (30g)	140	21	0.5	11	1	6
Angel Food Cake	1 slice (28g)	72	16	0	14	1.4	0.2
White Crackers	10 crackers (15g)	80	10	0	0	1	2
Instant Noodles	1 cup cooked	220	40	2	2	5	10
Rice Pudding	1/2 cup (113g)	150	30	0	14	3.5	3
Soft Drink Powder (with sugar)	1 tbsp (22g)	80	20	0	20	0	0
Fried Dough	1 piece (60g)	200	25	1	10	3	10
Cereal Bars	1 bar (30g)	120	24	1	12	2	3
Milkshake (vanilla)	1 small (12 fl oz)	360	52	0	44	8	10
Sweetened Iced Tea	1 cup (240ml)	90	22	0	22	0	0

Chocolate Pudding	1/2 cup (113g)	160	26	1	22	3	4.5
Fruit Pie Filling	1/3 cup (85g)	100	25	1	21	0	0
Canned Fruit in Heavy Syrup	1/2 cup (122g)	100	26	1	25	0	0
Glazed Doughnut	1 medium (64g)	240	30	1	10	4	12
Bagel (white)	1 large (100g)	250	50	2	5	10	1.5
Pita Bread (white)	1 large (60g)	165	33	1	0	5.5	0.7
Tortilla (flour)	1 medium (26g)	85	14	0.9	0.3	2.3	2.2
Syrup (corn)	2 tbsp (30ml)	120	30	0	30	0	0
Chocolate Bar (milk)	1 bar (44g)	230	26	1	24	3	13
Energy Drinks	1 can (250ml)	110	28	0	27	0.5	0.3
Flavored Milk (chocolate)	1 cup (240ml)	208	26	0	24	8	8
Sweet Corn (canned)	1/2 cup (128g)	90	22	2	4	2.5	1
Biscuits (sweet)	2 biscuits (30g)	140	20	0.5	7	2	6
Granola (sweetened)	1/2 cup (45g)	200	32	3	12	4	7
Chocolate Chip Cookies	4 cookies (56g)	280	38	2	24	3	14

Fruit Snacks	1 pouch (23g)	80	19	0	11	1	0
BBQ Sauce	2 tbsp (30ml)	60	14	0	10	0	0
Ketchup	1 tbsp (17g)	20	5	0	4	0	0
Teriyaki Sauce	1 tbsp (15ml)	15	3	0	3	1	0
Sweet Pickles	1 medium (23g)	30	7	0	7	0	0
Canned Baked Beans (sweetened)	1/2 cup (130g)	120	27	5	12	5	0.5
Fruit Flavored Yogurt	1 cup (245g)	230	42	0	38	10	3
Instant Pudding	1/2 cup prepared	140	30	0	24	0	3.5
Jellied Cranberry Sauce	1/4 cup (70g)	110	28	0	24	0	0
Sweetened Applesauce	1/2 cup (122g)	90	23	1.5	20	0	0
Caramel Sauce	2 tbsp (30ml)	103	17	0	15	0.5	2.3
Maltose	1 tbsp (20g)	60	15	0	15	0	0
Fruit Cocktail (light syrup)	1/2 cup (122g)	70	18	1	17	0	0
Sweetened Condensed Milk	1 oz (28g)	123	21	0	21	3	3.2
White Chocolate	1 oz (28g)	153	17	0	17	1.7	9
Marshmallow Fluff	2 tbsp (12g)	40	10	0	9	0	0

Frosted Flakes Cereal	3/4 cup (29g)	110	27	0	10	1	0
Grits (instant)	1 cup prepared	182	38	2	0	4	1
Pretzel Sticks	1 oz (28g)	109	23	1	1	2.6	0.8
Cinnamon Roll	1 small (60g)	223	30	1	15	4	9
Fruit Danish	1 piece (71g)	263	34	1	16	4	13
Sugar-Sweetened Gelatin	1/2 cup prepared	80	19	0	18	2	0
Hard Candy	3 pieces (18g)	70	18	0	11	0	0
Fudge	1 piece (28g)	90	18	0	16	1	2

Trans Fats and Saturated Fats

Trans fats, the true villains in the world of dietary fats, have a notorious reputation for a good reason. These fats are primarily created through an industrial process called hydrogenation, which turns liquid oils into solid fats. Think margarine and shortening, ingredients often found in processed foods, baked goods, and fried items.

The issue with trans fats lies in their ability to wreak havoc on our health. They've been linked to increased levels of bad cholesterol (LDL) and decreased levels of good cholesterol (HDL), significantly raising the risk of heart disease and stroke. Moreover, trans fats can contribute to inflammation, a root cause of many chronic diseases, and even insulin resistance, which is particularly concerning for those of us trying to manage our weight and metabolic health.

For someone following a metabolic confusion diet, the message is clear: trans fats are not your friends. Steering clear of processed foods and reading labels carefully can help you avoid these unwelcome guests.

Saturated fats have been at the center of dietary debates for decades, cast in a role that's both hero and villain. Found in animal products like meat and dairy, as well as tropical oils, saturated fats were once thought to be a leading cause of heart disease. Recent research, however, has started to paint a more nuanced picture, suggesting that the relationship between saturated fats and heart health might not be as straightforward as once believed.

In moderation, saturated fats can play a part in a balanced diet. They're essential for building cell membranes and producing certain hormones. The key, especially within the metabolic confusion framework, is balance and moderation. Including sources of saturated fats in your diet, like lean meats, dairy, and coconut oil, can be beneficial, as long as they are part of a diverse intake of fats that includes plenty of unsaturated fats from sources like fish, nuts, and seeds.

When it comes to trans fats and saturated fats, the strategy is simple: minimize and moderate. Completely avoiding trans fats is a wise move for anyone concerned about their health and metabolic efficiency. As for saturated fats, including them as part of a varied diet, balanced with a higher intake of unsaturated fats, can support your health goals without steering you off course.

Food	Portion Size	Trans Fats (g)	Saturated Fats (g)
Margarine (stick)	1 tbsp	1.6	2.1
Shortening	1 tbsp	1.7	3.2
Fried Chicken	1 piece	Varied	3-5
French Fries	1 medium serving	Varied	3.5
Doughnuts	1 medium	0.3-5	4.9
Cream-filled Pastries	1 medium	Varied	5-10
Butter	1 tbsp	0	7.2
Cheese (Cheddar)	1 oz	0	6

Pizza	1 slice	Varied	4-5
Ice Cream	1/2 cup	0.2	4.5
Processed Meat (Sausages)	2 links	Varied	7-10
Bacon	2 slices	0	3.8
Beef Ribs	3 oz	0	9
Pork Chops	3 oz	0	8.2
Lamb	3 oz	0	8
Coconut Oil	1 tbsp	0	11.2
Palm Oil	1 tbsp	0	7
Cream Cheese	1 oz	0	5
Sour Cream	1 tbsp	0	1.5
Milk Chocolate	1 oz	0	5
Lard	1 tbsp	0	5
Fast Food Burgers	1 medium burger	Varied	10-15
Potato Chips	1 oz (about 15 chips)	Varied	2-3
Microwave Popcorn	1 bag	Varied	5-6
Canned Frosting	2 tbsp	1.5	2.5
Packaged Cookies	4 cookies	Varied	3-4
Frozen Pizzas	1/4 pizza	Varied	5-6
Canned Soup (Cream-based)	1 cup	Varied	3-5

Meat Pies	1 medium pie	Varied	10-20
Chicken Nuggets	6 nuggets	Varied	2-3
Crackers (Butter-flavored)	5 crackers	Varied	2-3
Non-dairy Whipped Topping	2 tbsp	0.5	1.5
Heavy Cream	1 tbsp	0	3.5
Fatty Cuts of Beef	3 oz	0	5-7
Fatty Cuts of Pork	3 oz	0	5-7
Dark Chocolate	1 oz	0	5
Biscuits	1 medium	Varied	3-5
Cheesecake	1 slice	0	18
Croissants	1 medium	0	12
Puff Pastry	1 oz	Varied	5-6
Quiche	1 slice	Varied	10-15
Gravy (Cream-based)	1/4 cup	Varied	3-5
Full-fat Yogurt	1 cup	0	5
Tallow	1 tbsp	0	6.7
Ghee	1 tbsp	0	7.9
Fried Seafood	3 oz	Varied	3-7
Cream-filled Candy	1 oz	Varied	3-5
Butter-flavored Microwave Popcorn	1 bag	Varied	5-6

Snack Cakes	1 cake	Varied	5-10
Artificial Creamer	1 tbsp	0.1	0.5
Store-bought Pie	1 slice (1/8 of a 9" pie)	Varied	5-10
Fried Dough	1 medium piece	Varied	5-8
Commercially Baked Muffins	1 medium	Varied	5-7
Deep-fried Vegetables	1 cup	Varied	3-5
Cheese Dip	1/4 cup	Varied	5-7
Cream-based Salad Dressings	2 tbsp	Varied	2-4
Flavored Coffee Creamers	1 tbsp	0.1	1-2
Butter-flavored Syrup	2 tbsp	Varied	0-1
Commercially Prepared Biscuits	1 large	Varied	5-8
Chocolate Pudding	1/2 cup	0	3-5
Canned Chili Con Carne	1 cup	Varied	5-7
Boxed Macaroni and Cheese	1 cup prepared	Varied	3-5
Packaged Snack Cakes and Pastries	1 package	Varied	5-10
Fast Food Milkshakes	12 oz (small)	Varied	10-15
Commercially Prepared Fried Fish	1 piece	Varied	3-5
Store-bought Granola Bars	1 bar	Varied	2-3
Canned Coconut Milk	1 cup	0	21-24

Store-bought Frosting	2 tbsp	1.5	2.5
Pre-packaged Sandwiches	1 sandwich	Varied	5-10
Fast Food Onion Rings	1 medium order	Varied	3-5
Packaged Pie Crusts	1/8 crust	Varied	2-4
Store-bought Cheesecake	1 slice	Varied	10-15
Canned Biscuits and Rolls	1 biscuit/roll	Varied	2-5
Pre-made Cookie Dough	1 oz	Varied	2-3
Fast Food Taco Salad	1 salad	Varied	10-15
Store-bought Pound Cake	1 slice	Varied	5-7
Pre-packaged Frozen Meals	1 meal	Varied	5-10
Deli Meat	2 oz	Varied	2-5
Cured Meats (e.g., Salami, Pepperoni)	2 slices	Varied	3-5
Commercially Prepared Lasagna	1 cup	Varied	5-10
Fast Food Breakfast Sandwiches	1 sandwich	Varied	5-10
Store-bought Tiramisu	1 slice	Varied	10-12
Pre-made Cake Mixes	1/10 cake	Varied	2-5
Chocolate Bars (Milk Chocolate)	1 oz	0	5-7
Flavored Yogurts (with added sugar)	1 cup	0	3-5

Store-bought Scones	1 medium	Varied	5-8
Pre-packaged Quiche	1 slice	Varied	10-15
Fast Food Fried Shrimp	1 small order	Varied	3-5
Store-bought Layer Cakes	1 slice	Varied	10-15
Fast Food Chicken Tenders	3 pieces	Varied	2-4
Pre-packaged Croissant Sandwiches	1 sandwich	Varied	7-10
Store-bought Danish Pastries	1 pastry	Varied	5-7
Fast Food Sausage Pizza	1 slice (1/8 pizza)	Varied	5-8
Commercially Prepared Meatloaf	1 slice	Varied	5-10
Fast Food Cream Soups	1 cup	Varied	5-10
Pre-made Alfredo Sauce	1/2 cup	Varied	5-8
Store-bought Pecan Pie	1 slice	Varied	9-12
Fast Food Chili	1 cup	Varied	5-7
Pre-packaged Breakfast Pastries	1 pastry	Varied	5-7
Store-bought Flan	1/2 cup	Varied	3-5

It's important to note that "Varied" indicates that the trans fat content can vary based on the brand, preparation method, and serving size. Always check the nutrition labels for the most accurate information.

SAMPLE MEAL PLANS

14-Day High-Calorie Phase Meal Plan

Week 1

Day 1:

- Breakfast: Oatmeal with almond butter, banana slices, and a sprinkle of chia seeds.
- Snack: Greek yogurt with mixed berries and a drizzle of honey.
- Lunch: Quinoa salad with grilled chicken, avocado, black beans, corn, and a cilantro-lime dressing.
- Snack: A handful of almonds and a slice of whole-grain bread with avocado.
- Dinner: Baked salmon with sweet potato wedges and steamed broccoli.

Day 2:

- Breakfast: Whole grain pancakes topped with fresh strawberries and a dollop of ricotta cheese.
- Snack: Cottage cheese with pineapple chunks.
- Lunch: Turkey and avocado wrap with whole-grain tortilla, mixed greens, and tomato.
- Snack: Apple slices with peanut butter.
- Dinner: Stir-fried beef with bell peppers, onions, and brown rice.

Day 3:

- Breakfast: Scrambled eggs with spinach, feta cheese, and whole-grain toast.

- Snack: A smoothie made with kale, banana, protein powder, and almond milk.
- Lunch: Tuna salad with mixed greens, cherry tomatoes, olives, and a balsamic vinaigrette.
- Snack: Carrot sticks with hummus.
- Dinner: Chicken parmesan over whole wheat pasta with a side salad.

Day 4:

- Breakfast: Greek yogurt parfait with granola, mixed nuts, and honey.
- Snack: A pear and a handful of walnuts.
- Lunch: Grilled shrimp taco bowls with rice, black beans, avocado, salsa, and cheese.
- Snack: A protein bar and a banana.
- Dinner: Pork tenderloin with roasted Brussels sprouts and quinoa.

Day 5:

- Breakfast: Banana and almond butter smoothie with a scoop of protein powder.
- Snack: A hard-boiled egg and orange slices.
- Lunch: Spinach and goat cheese stuffed chicken breast with roasted sweet potatoes.
- Snack: A small bowl of mixed berries and a handful of pumpkin seeds.
- Dinner: Vegetarian chili with kidney beans, lentils, and a variety of vegetables, served with cornbread.

Day 6:

- Breakfast: French toast made with whole-grain bread, topped with blueberries and maple syrup.
- Snack: A slice of cantaloupe and cottage cheese.
- Lunch: Beef and vegetable stir-fry with brown rice.
- Snack: A handful of mixed nuts and a kiwi.
- Dinner: Baked cod with a lemon-butter sauce, asparagus, and wild rice.

Day 7:

- Breakfast: A smoothie bowl with acai, bananas, mixed berries, granola, and coconut flakes.
- Snack: Sliced cucumber and cherry tomatoes with a tzatziki dip.
- Lunch: Roast beef sandwich on whole-grain bread with lettuce, tomato, and mustard, served with a side of kale chips.
- Snack: Dark chocolate (a small piece) and a handful of raspberries.
- Dinner: Grilled lamb chops with mint pesto, roasted potatoes, and green beans.

Day 8:

- **Breakfast:** Chia pudding made with coconut milk, topped with mango and coconut flakes.
- **Lunch:** Steak salad with mixed greens, blue cheese, walnuts, and a balsamic vinaigrette.
- **Dinner:** Roasted duck breast with wild rice and a cherry sauce, served with steamed green beans.
- **Snacks:** A peach; whole-grain toast with ricotta and honey.

Day 9:

- **Breakfast:** Breakfast burrito with scrambled eggs, chorizo, potatoes, cheese, and salsa wrapped in a whole-grain tortilla.
- **Lunch:** Soba noodle bowl with tofu, edamame, carrots, bell peppers, and a peanut sauce.
- **Dinner:** Grilled swordfish with a lemon-herb dressing, served with a couscous salad.
- **Snacks:** A handful of dried fruit and nuts; Greek yogurt with mixed berries.

Day 10:

- **Breakfast:** Baked avocado eggs, with a side of whole-grain toast and a tomato salad.
- **Lunch:** Chicken Caesar wrap with whole-grain tortilla, romaine lettuce, Parmesan cheese, and Caesar dressing.
- **Dinner:** Pork loin roast with apple sauce, served with roasted sweet potatoes and asparagus.
- **Snacks:** Cottage cheese with sliced peaches; a granola bar.

Day 11:

- **Breakfast:** Smoothie with kale, avocado, banana, protein powder, and almond milk.
- **Lunch:** Quiche with a mixed green salad on the side.
- **Dinner:** Beef stroganoff over whole-wheat egg noodles, served with sautéed spinach.
- **Snacks:** Almond butter on whole-grain crackers; a kiwi.

Day 12:

- **Breakfast:** Whole grain waffles with peanut butter, banana slices, and a sprinkle of chia seeds.

- **Lunch:** Mediterranean chickpea salad with tomatoes, cucumber, olives, feta, and a lemon-olive oil dressing.
- **Dinner:** Baked cod with a herb crust, served with mashed potatoes and steamed broccoli.
- **Snacks:** A protein shake; celery sticks with cream cheese.

Day 13:

- **Breakfast:** Granola with milk, topped with sliced strawberries and a drizzle of honey.
- **Lunch:** Turkey and cranberry sauce sandwich on whole-grain bread, with a side of sweet potato fries.
- **Dinner:** Spaghetti Carbonara with a side of arugula and cherry tomato salad.
- **Snacks:** An orange; a handful of pumpkin seeds.

Day 14:

- **Breakfast:** Omelet with mushrooms, onions, bell peppers, and cheese, served with whole-grain toast.
- **Lunch:** Grilled vegetable and hummus wrap in a whole-grain tortilla, with a side of Greek yogurt.
- **Dinner:** Moroccan lamb tagine with apricots and almonds, served over couscous.
- **Snacks:** A banana; rice cakes with avocado.

14-Day Low-Calorie Phase Meal Plan

Day 1:

- **Breakfast:** Scrambled eggs with spinach and tomatoes.
- **Lunch:** Mixed green salad with grilled chicken breast, cucumber, and a lemon vinaigrette.
- **Dinner:** Baked cod with steamed green beans and quinoa.

Day 2:

- **Breakfast:** Greek yogurt with a handful of berries and a sprinkle of flaxseeds.
- **Lunch:** Lentil soup with a side of mixed greens.
- **Dinner:** Stir-fried tofu with broccoli, bell pepper, and a side of cauliflower rice.

Day 3:

- **Breakfast:** Oatmeal topped with sliced apple and cinnamon.
- **Lunch:** Turkey and avocado wrap with whole wheat tortilla and side salad.
- **Dinner:** Grilled shrimp over a bed of zucchini noodles and marinara sauce.

Day 4:

- **Breakfast:** Smoothie made with spinach, banana, almond milk, and protein powder.
- **Lunch:** Quinoa and black bean salad with corn, tomatoes, and cilantro.
- **Dinner:** Chicken fajitas with sautéed onions and peppers, served without the tortillas.

Day 5:

- **Breakfast:** Cottage cheese with pineapple chunks.
- **Lunch:** Vegetable stir-fry with a small portion of brown rice.
- **Dinner:** Baked salmon with asparagus and a side of mixed leafy greens.

Day 6:

- **Breakfast:** Boiled eggs and a side of grapefruit.
- **Lunch:** Chickpea salad with cucumbers, tomatoes, feta, and olives.
- **Dinner:** Turkey meatballs with spaghetti squash and a side of steamed broccoli.

Day 7:

- **Breakfast:** Protein pancakes topped with a small amount of natural peanut butter and strawberries.
- **Lunch:** Tuna salad stuffed in bell peppers.
- **Dinner:** Grilled chicken with roasted Brussels sprouts and a small baked sweet potato.

Day 8:

- **Breakfast:** Chia seed pudding made with almond milk and topped with kiwi.
- **Lunch:** Sliced beef and avocado salad with a sprinkle of sesame seeds and soy sauce dressing.
- **Dinner:** Zucchini lasagna with ground turkey and low-fat ricotta cheese.

Day 9:

- **Breakfast:** Green smoothie with kale, apple, cucumber, and ginger.

- **Lunch:** Cauliflower rice and vegetable stir-fry with a few pieces of baked tofu.
- **Dinner:** Grilled pork chop with a side of apple slaw.

Day 10:

- **Breakfast:** Berry and spinach smoothie with a scoop of protein powder.
- **Lunch:** Roasted vegetable salad with mixed greens, goat cheese, and balsamic vinaigrette.
- **Dinner:** Lemon garlic tilapia with a side of roasted cauliflower.

Day 11:

- **Breakfast:** Egg white omelet with mushrooms, onions, and spinach.
- **Lunch:** Chicken Caesar salad with a low-calorie dressing.
- **Dinner:** Beef and vegetable skewers with a side of cucumber salad.

Day 12:

- **Breakfast:** Overnight oats made with almond milk, chia seeds, and topped with raspberries.
- **Lunch:** Sardine salad with mixed greens, tomatoes, and a lemon olive oil dressing.
- **Dinner:** Stuffed bell peppers with ground chicken, tomatoes, and a small amount of quinoa.

Day 13:

- **Breakfast:** A slice of whole-grain toast with avocado and poached egg.
- **Lunch:** Broccoli and almond soup with a side of kale salad.

- **Dinner:** Baked haddock with a side of sautéed spinach and garlic.

Day 14:

- **Breakfast:** Smoothie bowl with mixed berries, spinach, and a sprinkle of nuts.
- **Lunch:** Quinoa salad with cucumber, cherry tomatoes, and grilled halloumi cheese.
- **Dinner:** Grilled vegetable platter with a small portion of grilled chicken breast.

Tips for Meal Planning and Preparation

Embarking on a journey with the metabolic confusion diet, especially for endomorph women, requires not just commitment but also a strategic approach to meal planning and preparation. This process can seem daunting at first, but with the right tips and techniques, it becomes not only manageable but also enjoyable, turning into a habit that supports your health and fitness goals in the long run. Let's dive into some essential tips for meal planning and preparation that can make your journey smoother and more effective.

1. Understand Your Nutritional Needs

Before anything else, it's crucial to have a clear understanding of your nutritional needs. This means knowing the balance of macronutrients (proteins, carbohydrates, and fats) that work best for your body type and the goals you're aiming to achieve with the metabolic confusion diet. Remember, what works for someone else might not work for you, so tailor your plan to meet your unique requirements.

2. Start with a Plan

- **Set Your Goals:** Clearly define what you want to achieve with your meal plan. Are you looking to lose weight, gain muscle, or simply maintain a healthy lifestyle? Your goals will significantly influence your approach to meal planning.

- **Create a Meal Calendar:** Dedicate some time each week to map out your meals and snacks. This includes high-calorie and low-calorie days if you're following a metabolic confusion diet. Planning ahead prevents last-minute unhealthy choices.

- **Incorporate Variety:** To prevent boredom and ensure a wide range of nutrients, include a variety of foods in your plan. Experiment with different cuisines and flavors to keep things interesting.

3. Smart Grocery Shopping

- **Make a List:** Based on your meal plan, create a detailed shopping list. This keeps you focused and helps avoid impulse buys that might not fit into your diet.

- **Shop the Perimeter:** Most grocery stores are designed with fresh produce, meats, and dairy around the perimeter. Stick to these areas to fill your cart with whole foods.

- **Consider Bulk Buying:** For non-perishable items and staples like rice, beans, and frozen vegetables, buying in bulk can save time and money.

4. Preparation is Key

- **Batch Cooking:** Dedicate a few hours each week to cook large batches of staples like grains, proteins, and vegetables. This makes assembling meals throughout the week quick and easy.

- **Portion and Store:** Divide cooked foods into portion-controlled containers. This not only helps with portion control but also makes grabbing a meal on-the-go hassle-free.
- **Freeze for Later:** Not all meals need to be eaten within the week. Freezing portions can be a lifesaver for busy weeks ahead or when you need a break from cooking.

5. Keep Snacks Simple and Healthy

- **Prep Snacks in Advance:** Just like meals, having ready-to-eat snacks can prevent reaching for unhealthy options. Think cut vegetables, fruits, nuts, and yogurt.
- **Portion Control:** Even healthy snacks can contribute to calorie overload if not managed. Keep an eye on portion sizes, especially on low-calorie days.

6. Embrace Flexibility

- **Be Ready to Swap:** Sometimes, life happens, and you might not stick to your meal plan 100%. Having a flexible mindset allows you to swap meals around as needed without feeling like you've failed.
- **Listen to Your Body:** Some days you might feel more hungry or less interested in certain foods. It's okay to adjust your plan based on your body's signals, as long as you stay within your nutritional goals.

7. Make It Enjoyable

- **Involve Family or Friends:** Meal planning and cooking don't have to be solitary tasks. Involve your loved ones to make it a fun and engaging activity.

- **Try New Recipes:** Regularly introduce new recipes to keep your diet exciting and to challenge your culinary skills.

- **Celebrate Small Wins:** Successfully sticking to your meal plan, trying a new vegetable, or mastering a recipe are all achievements worth celebrating.

8. Use Technology to Your Advantage

- **Meal Planning Apps:** Numerous apps can help with meal planning, grocery shopping, and even tracking your nutritional intake. Find one that suits your needs.

- **Online Resources:** There's a wealth of information online, from recipes to nutritional advice. Use these resources to inspire and educate yourself further.

9. Stay Hydrated

- **Water First:** Before reaching for a snack, drink a glass of water. Thirst is often mistaken for hunger.

- **Incorporate into Your Plan:** Just as you plan your meals, plan your water intake to ensure you're staying adequately hydrated throughout the day.

CONCLUSION AND MOVING FORWARD

Embarking on the metabolic confusion diet represents a transformative journey towards health, wellness, and understanding your body's unique needs. This journey, marked by its phases of high and low caloric intake, aims not only to enhance your metabolism but also to redefine your relationship with food. As we navigate through this pathway, it's essential to distill the experiences, lessons, and outcomes into key takeaways, strategies for maintaining long-term results, and sources of motivation for a continued health and wellness journey.

Key Takeaways from the Metabolic Confusion Diet

Understanding Your Body's Needs: One of the most profound lessons from the metabolic confusion diet is the importance of tuning in to your body's signals. This diet teaches you that your metabolic rate is not static; it can be influenced by dietary patterns, physical activity, and even the types of food you consume. Learning to listen to your body's cues for hunger, fullness, and energy levels is crucial.

Flexibility and Adaptability: The metabolic confusion diet highlights the power of flexibility in your eating habits. By alternating between high-calorie and low-calorie days, you learn that strict, monotonous dieting is not the only path to weight loss and health. This adaptability can be a liberating discovery, making it easier to stick with your diet and make adjustments as needed.

Nutrient Density Over Calorie Counting: While the diet does involve a level of calorie awareness, it emphasizes the quality of the calories you consume. Nutrient-dense foods—rich in vitamins, minerals, fiber, and other essential nutrients—take precedence, teaching you to make smarter food choices that support your overall health, beyond just weight management.

Metabolism is Modifiable: A pivotal realization from following the metabolic confusion diet is that your metabolism is not fixed. You have the power to influence and improve it through dietary choices, timing, and physical activity. This understanding can be incredibly empowering, offering hope and motivation to those who may have felt stuck or defeated by previous weight loss attempts.

How to Maintain Results Long-Term

Establishing a Balanced Diet: Long-term success with the metabolic confusion diet—or any diet, for that matter—relies on finding a balanced approach to eating that can be sustained indefinitely. Incorporate a wide variety of foods from all food groups to ensure you're getting a comprehensive array of nutrients. Avoid extreme restrictions or the elimination of entire food categories, which can lead to nutritional deficiencies and disordered eating patterns.

Regular Physical Activity: Exercise is a cornerstone of maintaining the results achieved through the metabolic confusion diet. Find activities you enjoy and can commit to regularly, whether it's walking, cycling, strength training, yoga, or a combination of several. Exercise not only helps in maintaining weight but also boosts your mood, improves sleep quality, and increases energy levels.

Mindful Eating Practices: Cultivating mindfulness around food and eating habits can significantly contribute to long-term success. Pay attention to your body's hunger and satiety signals, eat slowly, and savor your food. This practice can help prevent overeating and promote a healthier relationship with food.

Continual Learning and Adaptation: As you progress on your health journey, your body's needs may change. Stay open to learning and adapting your dietary approach as necessary. This might mean adjusting your caloric intake, experimenting with different macronutrient ratios, or introducing new foods and recipes to keep things interesting.

Encouragement for Continued Health and Wellness Journey

Celebrate Your Progress: Remember to celebrate the milestones you've achieved, no matter how small they may seem. Every step forward is a testament to your commitment, resilience, and dedication to your health. Celebrations can be simple, like treating yourself to a new book, taking a day off for self-care, or enjoying a special meal with loved ones.

Seek Support and Community: You don't have to walk this path alone. Seek support from friends, family, or online communities who share your health and wellness goals. Sharing experiences, challenges, and successes can provide motivation, accountability, and a sense of belonging.

Stay Curious and Open to New Experiences: Health and wellness are ongoing journeys with no final destination. Stay curious and open to trying new foods, fitness routines, and wellness practices. This openness can lead to discoveries that further enrich your life and contribute to your well-being.

Remember Your 'Why': On days when motivation wanes, remind yourself why you started this journey. Whether it's improving your health, feeling more energetic, or setting a good example for your family, your "why" can serve as a powerful motivator to keep moving forward.

Be Kind to Yourself: Finally, practice self-compassion on your journey. There will be setbacks and challenges, but they do not define your worth or your progress. Treat yourself with kindness, patience, and understanding, just as you would a dear friend.

BONUS: SMOOTHIE RECIPES FOR WEIGHT LOSS

Green Detox Smoothie

A refreshing and cleansing drink packed with antioxidants and fiber to kickstart your metabolism and aid in digestion.

Prep Time: 5 minutes Cooking Time: 0 minutes Serving Size: 1 serving

Ingredients:

- 1 cup spinach leaves
- 1/2 green apple, sliced
- 1/2 banana
- 1 tablespoon chia seeds
- 1 cup unsweetened almond milk
- 1 teaspoon fresh ginger, grated
- Ice cubes (optional)

Instructions:

1. Combine spinach, green apple, banana, chia seeds, almond milk, and fresh ginger in a blender.
2. Blend until smooth. Add ice cubes if you prefer a colder smoothie.
3. Serve immediately for the best taste and nutrient retention.

Nutritional Information (per serving):

- Calories: 180
- Protein: 4g
- Carbohydrates: 33g

- Dietary Fiber: 8g
- Fat: 4g
- Saturated Fat: 0.5g
- Sodium: 180mg
- Potassium: 500mg

Berry Protein Power Smoothie

A protein-packed smoothie that keeps you full for hours. Berries add natural sweetness and a load of antioxidants.

Prep Time: 5 minutes Cooking Time: 0 minutes Serving Size: 1 serving

Ingredients:

- 1/2 cup mixed berries (blueberries, strawberries, raspberries)
- 1 scoop vanilla whey protein powder
- 1 tablespoon flaxseed meal
- 1 cup unsweetened almond milk
- Ice cubes (optional)

Instructions:

1. Place the mixed berries, whey protein powder, flaxseed meal, and almond milk into a blender.
2. Blend until smooth. For a thicker smoothie, add ice cubes and blend again.
3. Enjoy immediately to maximize the benefits of the protein and fiber.

Nutritional Information (per serving):

- Calories: 220
- Protein: 25g

- Carbohydrates: 18g

- Dietary Fiber: 5g

- Fat: 6g

- Saturated Fat: 0.5g

- Sodium: 190mg

- Potassium: 300mg

Tropical Turmeric Cleanser Smoothie

This smoothie combines the anti-inflammatory benefits of turmeric with the tropical flavors of mango and pineapple.

Prep Time: 5 minutes Cooking Time: 0 minutes Serving Size: 1 serving

Ingredients:

- 1 cup frozen mango chunks

- 1/2 cup pineapple chunks

- 1/2 teaspoon ground turmeric

- 1 tablespoon hemp seeds

- 1 cup coconut water

- Ice cubes (optional)

Instructions:

1. Blend the mango, pineapple, turmeric, hemp seeds, and coconut water until smooth.

2. Add ice cubes for a refreshing chill, if desired.

3. Serve fresh to enjoy its vibrant flavors and nutritional benefits.

Nutritional Information (per serving):

- Calories: 180

- Protein: 3g

- Carbohydrates: 36g

- Dietary Fiber: 4g

- Fat: 4g

- Saturated Fat: 0.5g

- Sodium: 60mg

- Potassium: 500mg

Cinnamon Almond Joy Smoothie

A delightful smoothie that mimics the flavors of an almond joy candy bar, without the guilt. Cinnamon regulates blood sugar levels.

Prep Time: 5 minutes Cooking Time: 0 minutes Serving Size: 1 serving

Ingredients:

- 1 banana

- 1 tablespoon almond butter

- 1 tablespoon unsweetened cocoa powder

- 1/2 teaspoon ground cinnamon

- 1 cup unsweetened almond milk

- Ice cubes (optional)

Instructions:

1. Blend the banana, almond butter, cocoa powder, cinnamon, and almond milk until smooth.

2. Add ice to reach desired consistency and blend again.

3. Enjoy this guilt-free treat immediately.

Nutritional Information (per serving):

- Calories: 220

- Protein: 5g

- Carbohydrates: 30g
- Dietary Fiber: 7g
- Fat: 11g
- Saturated Fat: 1g
- Sodium: 180mg
- Potassium: 450mg

Avocado & Mint Refresh Smoothie

A creamy and refreshing smoothie, perfect for hot days. Avocado provides healthy fats and fiber for fullness.

Prep Time: 5 minutes Cooking Time: 0 minutes Serving Size: 1 serving

Ingredients:

- 1/2 ripe avocado
- 1/2 cup spinach leaves
- 10 mint leaves
- 1/2 cucumber, sliced
- 1 tablespoon lime juice
- 1 cup unsweetened almond milk
- Ice cubes (optional)

Instructions:

1. Combine avocado, spinach, mint, cucumber, lime juice, and almond milk in a blender.
2. Blend until creamy. Add ice for a cooler smoothie.
3. Serve immediately to enjoy its freshness and creamy texture.

Nutritional Information (per serving):

- Calories: 190

- Protein: 3g

- Carbohydrates: 15g

- Dietary Fiber: 7g

- Fat: 14g

- Saturated Fat: 2g

- Sodium: 180mg

- Potassium: 550mg

Peanut Butter Berry Protein Smoothie

A delightful blend of berries and peanut butter, offering a satisfying mix of protein and fiber to keep you full.

Prep Time: 5 minutes Cooking Time: 0 minutes Serving Size: 1 serving

Ingredients:

- 1/2 cup frozen mixed berries

- 1 tablespoon natural peanut butter

- 1 scoop vanilla or berry protein powder

- 1 cup unsweetened almond milk

- Ice cubes (optional)

Instructions:

1. Add the frozen berries, peanut butter, protein powder, and almond milk to a blender.

2. Blend until smooth. Add ice to achieve your desired consistency.

3. Drink immediately to enjoy the creamy, rich flavors.

Nutritional Information (per serving):

- Calories: 280

- Protein: 28g

- Carbohydrates: 24g

- Dietary Fiber: 6g

- Fat: 10g

- Saturated Fat: 2g

- Sodium: 250mg

- Potassium: 400mg

Zesty Lemon Apple Smoothie

A refreshing and invigorating smoothie that combines the tanginess of lemon with the sweetness of apples.

Prep Time: 5 minutes Cooking Time: 0 minutes Serving Size: 1 serving

Ingredients:

- 1 green apple, cored and sliced

- Juice of 1 lemon

- 1/2 cucumber, sliced

- 1 tablespoon chia seeds

- 1 cup water or coconut water

- Ice cubes (optional)

Instructions:

1. Combine the apple, lemon juice, cucumber, chia seeds, and water in a blender.

2. Blend until smooth. Add ice for additional refreshment.

3. Serve immediately for a burst of zesty flavor.

Nutritional Information (per serving):

- Calories: 150

- Protein: 3g
- Carbohydrates: 30g
- Dietary Fiber: 8g
- Fat: 3g
- Saturated Fat: 0g
- Sodium: 20mg
- Potassium: 400mg

Spiced Carrot Cake Smoothie

Enjoy the comforting taste of carrot cake in a healthy, drinkable form, complete with the nutritional benefits of carrots and spices.

Prep Time: 5 minutes Cooking Time: 0 minutes Serving Size: 1 serving

Ingredients:

- 1 large carrot, peeled and chopped
- 1/4 cup rolled oats
- 1 tablespoon walnuts
- 1/2 teaspoon cinnamon
- Pinch of nutmeg
- 1 cup unsweetened almond milk
- 1 teaspoon maple syrup (optional)
- Ice cubes (optional)

Instructions:

1. Place the carrot, oats, walnuts, cinnamon, nutmeg, almond milk, and maple syrup into a blender.
2. Blend until smooth. Add ice to reach your preferred temperature.

3. Pour into a glass and enjoy this guilt-free treat.

Nutritional Information (per serving):

- Calories: 220
- Protein: 5g
- Carbohydrates: 35g
- Dietary Fiber: 7g
- Fat: 7g
- Saturated Fat: 0.5g
- Sodium: 180mg
- Potassium: 450mg

Cooling Mint Cucumber Smoothie

A hydrating and cooling smoothie perfect for hot days, combining the freshness of mint and cucumber.

Prep Time: 5 minutes Cooking Time: 0 minutes Serving Size: 1 serving

Ingredients:

- 1 cup cucumber, sliced
- 1/2 cup fresh mint leaves
- 1/2 lime, juiced
- 1 tablespoon honey or agave nectar
- 1 cup water or coconut water
- Ice cubes (optional)

Instructions:

1. Blend cucumber, mint leaves, lime juice, honey, and water until smooth.
2. Add ice to the blender for a colder beverage if desired.

3. Enjoy immediately for a refreshing, hydrating experience.

Nutritional Information (per serving):

- Calories: 100
- Protein: 1g
- Carbohydrates: 25g
- Dietary Fiber: 2g
- Fat: 0g
- Saturated Fat: 0g
- Sodium: 20mg
- Potassium: 300mg

BONUS: WORKBOOK FOR METABOLIC CONFUSION ACTIVITIES

Metabolic Confusion Meal Planner Worksheet

Name: _______________________________

Week Starting: ____________________

Phase: ☐ High-Calorie ☐ Low-Calorie

Daily Meal Plan

Day	Breakfast	Lunch	Dinner	Snacks
Monday				
Tuesday				
Wednesday				
Thursday				
Friday				

<table>
<tr><td>Saturday</td><td></td><td></td><td></td><td></td></tr>
<tr><td>Sunday</td><td></td><td></td><td></td><td></td></tr>
</table>

Notes and Adjustments:

Monday:

____

____

____

Tuesday:

____

____

____

Wednesday:

____

Thursday:

Friday:

Saturday:

Sunday:

____

____

____

Weekly Grocery List

Proteins:

____

____

____

Vegetables:

____

____

____

Fruits:

____

____

Carbs:

Fats:

Dairy:

Beverages:

115

Snacks:

Others:

Reflection:

What worked well this week?

____

____

____

Challenges faced:

____

____

____

Adjustments for next week:

____

____

____

Daily Nutrition and Activity Log

Date: _________

Nutrition Log

Meal Type	Food Item	Portion Size	Calories	Protein (g)	Carbs (g)	Fats (g)	Fiber (g)
Breakfast							
Lunch							
Dinner							
Snacks							

Total Daily Intake: Calories: ___________ Protein (g): ___________ Carbs (g): ___________ Fats (g): ___________ Fiber (g): ___________

Hydration Log

Time	Beverage	Quantity (ml)	Notes
Morning			
Noon			
Afternoon			
Evening			

Total Daily Fluid Intake: ___________ ml

Activity Log

Activity Type	Duration (min)	Intensity (Low/Medium/High)	Estimated Calories Burned	Notes
Cardio				
Strength Training				
Yoga/Stretching				
Other				

Total Daily Activity: _________ min

Total Calories Burned: _________

Reflections and Notes

- **Energy Levels Today (Low/Medium/High):** _________
- **Mood (Scale 1-10):** _________
- **Hunger Levels Before and After Meals (Scale 1-10):**
  ____
- **Overall Satisfaction with Meals (Scale 1-10):** _________

____

____

____

____

To use this log:

- **For the Nutrition Log**, list everything you eat and drink throughout the day. Use online resources or food labels to fill in the macronutrients and calorie content.

- **In the Hydration Log**, keep track of all fluids consumed, aiming for at least 8 glasses (about 2 liters) of water per day, unless otherwise advised by a healthcare provider.

- **For the Activity Log**, include all physical activities performed, estimating calories burned if possible. Use a fitness tracker or online calculators for more accurate estimates.

- **Under Reflections and Notes**, jot down how you felt throughout the day, how your meals and activities contributed to those feelings, and any other observations that might inform future changes to your diet or exercise plan.

Metabolic Confusion Phase Reflection Journal

Name: ________________________________

Date: ________________________________

Phase: (High-Calorie / Low-Calorie) (Circle One)

Duration of Phase: ________________________________ (e.g., 1 week, 2 weeks)

Daily Reflections

Day	Physical Energy Level	Hunger Level	Mood and Emotional State	Overall Satisfaction (1-10)	Notes and Observations
Day 1					
Day 2					
Day 3					
Day 4					
Day 5					
Day 6					
Day 7					

Physical Energy Level & Hunger Level: Use a scale from 1 (Very Low) to 10 (Very High).

Mood and Emotional State: Describe briefly (e.g., motivated, frustrated, energetic).

Overall Satisfaction: Rate your overall satisfaction with the phase on a scale from 1 (Not Satisfied) to 10 (Very Satisfied).

Challenges and Successes

- **What were the biggest challenges you faced during this phase?**

  ____

  ____

- **What successes or positive outcomes did you experience?**

  ____

  ____

Dietary Reflections

- **Were there any foods or meals that particularly helped or hindered your progress?**

  ____

  ____

- **How well did you stick to your planned meals and snacks? (1-10)**

  ____

Physical Activity

- **Describe your physical activity level and types of exercise during this phase:**

  ____

  ____

- **Did your exercise routine impact your energy levels or hunger? How?**

  ____

  ____

Adjustments for Next Phase

- **Based on your reflections, what adjustments will you make for the next phase?**

- **Are there any specific goals you want to set for the next phase?**

Additional Notes and Observations

This Metabolic Confusion Phase Reflection Journal serves as a comprehensive tool to monitor your journey, enabling you to make informed decisions and modifications to your diet and lifestyle for improved health and well-being. Regularly completing this journal can provide valuable insights into how different phases affect you physically and emotionally, guiding you toward a more personalized and effective approach to the metabolic confusion diet.

Grocery Shopping and Meal Prep Guide for Metabolic Confusion Diet

Part 1: Weekly Meal Planning

Instructions: Plan your meals for the week ahead, considering the phase you're in (high-calorie or low-calorie). Fill in the table with your chosen meals and snacks for each day.

Day	Breakfast	Lunch	Dinner	Snacks
Monday				
Tuesday				
Wednesday				
Thursday				
Friday				
Saturday				
Sunday				

Part 2: Grocery Shopping List

Instructions: Based on your meal plan, list the ingredients needed for the week. Organize your list by food categories to streamline your shopping experience.

- **Proteins:**
  - ☐ Chicken breast
  - ☐ Salmon
  - ☐ Tofu
  - ☐ Eggs
- **Vegetables:**
  - ☐ Spinach
  - ☐ Broccoli
  - ☐ Bell peppers
  - ☐ Sweet potatoes
- **Fruits:**
  - ☐ Berries
  - ☐ Apples
  - ☐ Bananas
- **Carbohydrates:**
  - ☐ Quinoa
  - ☐ Brown rice
  - ☐ Whole grain pasta

- [ ] Oats

- **Fats:**

  - [ ] Avocados

  - [ ] Olive oil

  - [ ] Almonds

  - [ ] Chia seeds

- **Dairy/Dairy Alternatives:**

  - [ ] Greek yogurt

  - [ ] Almond milk

  - [ ] Cheese

- **Miscellaneous:**

  - [ ] Spices & herbs

  - [ ] Condiments

  - [ ] Protein powder

Part 3: Meal Prep Task List

Instructions: Outline the meal prep tasks for your upcoming week. This can include washing and chopping vegetables, cooking grains in bulk, preparing proteins, or assembling meals.

Task	Day/Time	Notes
Prep chicken breast	Sunday, 3 PM	Marinate for Monday & Tuesday
Cook quinoa in bulk	Sunday, 4 PM	Store in fridge

Part 4: Reflection and Notes

Instructions: After completing your week, reflect on what worked well and what could be improved. Note any adjustments for next week's plan.

What meals were most enjoyable?

____

____

____

____

What prep tasks simplified your week?

____

____

____

____

Any ingredients you didn't use?

____

____

____

____

Adjustments for next week:

____

____

____

____

Progress Tracker and Goal Setting Worksheet

Personal Information

- Name: ___________________________________
- Start Date: ______________________________
- End Date (if applicable): _______________

Goal Setting

1. **Short-Term Goals** (Next 4 Weeks)

   - Goal 1:

     ____

     - Deadline: ___________________
   - Goal 2:

     ____

     - Deadline: ___________________
   - Goal 3:

     ____

     - Deadline: ___________________

2. **Long-Term Goals** (Next 3-6 Months)

   - Goal 1:

     ____

     - Deadline: ___________________
   - Goal 2:

     ____

     - Deadline: ___________________
   - Goal 3:

     ____

- Deadline: _______________________

Weekly Progress Tracker

Week	Date	Weight	High-Calorie Days	Low-Calorie Days	Exercise Completed	Overall Energy Level	Notes
1							
2							
3							
4							

Energy Level: Low = 1, High = 5

Achievements and Reflections

1. **This Week's Achievements:**

Achievement 1:

____

Achievement 2:

____

Achievement 3:

____

2. Challenges Faced:

Challenge 1:

____

Challenge 2:

____

Challenge 3:

____

3. Next Week's Focus:

Focus 1:

____

Focus 2:

____

Focus 3:

____

Goal Revision (If Needed)

- Revised Goal:

  ____

- Reason for Revision:

  ____

- New Deadline:

  ____

Notes

____

____

____

____

____